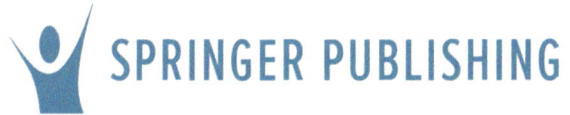
# SPRINGER PUBLISHING

AF132361

# GET THE MOST FROM YOUR BOOK

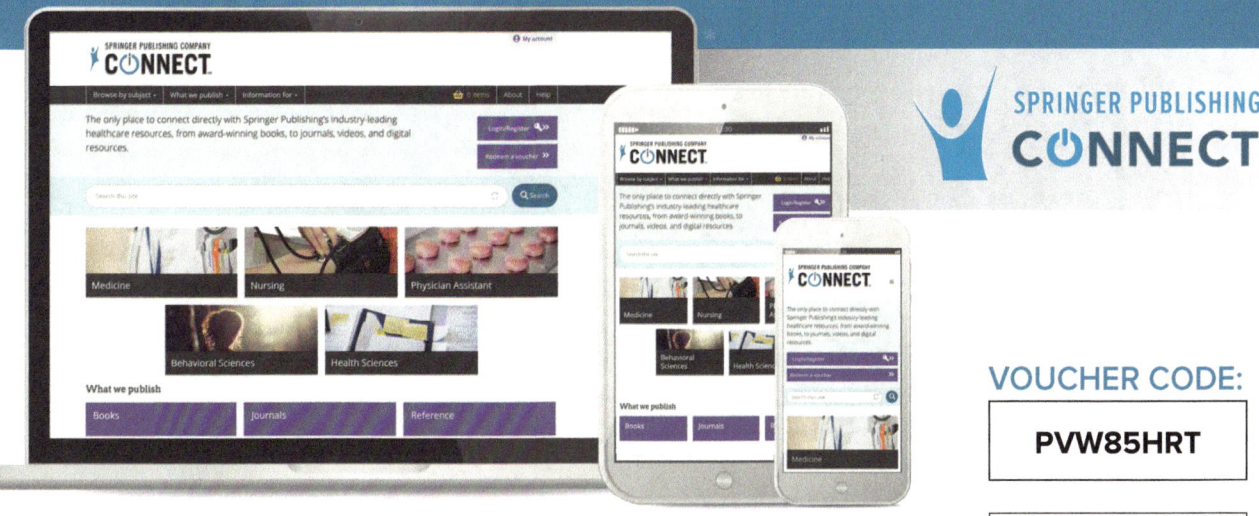

**VOUCHER CODE:**

**PVW85HRT**

## Online Access

Your print purchase of *Proposal Writing for the DNP Project,* Fourth Edition, includes **online access via Springer Publishing Connect™** to increase accessibility, portability, and searchability.

**Insert the code** at http://connect.springerpub.com/content/book/978-0-8261-8829-8 or scan the QR code and insert the voucher code today!

*Having trouble? Contact our customer service department at* **cs@springerpub.com**

## Instructor Resource Access for Adopters

**Let us do some of the heavy lifting to create an engaging classroom experience with a variety of instructor resources included in most textbooks SUCH AS:**

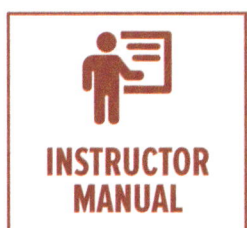

**INSTRUCTOR MANUAL**

**POWERPOINTS**

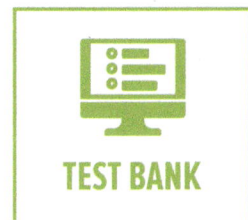

**TEST BANK**

Visit **https://connect.springerpub.com/** and look for the **"Show Supplementary"** button on your **book homepage** to see what is available to instructors! First time using Springer Publishing Connect?
Email **textbook@springerpub.com** to create an account and start unlocking valuable resources.

# Proposal Writing for the DNP Project

**Wanda Bonnel, PhD, APRN, ANEF,** is faculty emeritus at the University of Kansas School of Nursing, Kansas City, Kansas. She is a fellow of the National League for Nursing Academy and recipient of numerous awards, including both the Distinguished Nursing Alumna Award and the Chancellor's Distinguished Teaching Award at the University of Kansas. Dr. Bonnel has received multiple funded grants, including the Health Resources and Services Administration (HRSA) online Health Professions Educator Certificate program. She has published numerous peer-reviewed abstracts and articles in geriatric and educator specialty journals, including *Clinical Advisor* and *Journal of Professional Nursing*. In addition to this text, she coauthored the textbook *Teaching Technologies in Nursing and the Health Professions* (2019). As a specialist in geriatrics and nursing education, she has taught courses in master's, DNP, and doctoral programs, including advanced clinical residency and project courses for DNPs. Her ongoing research interests include online learning best practices and advanced practice mentoring.

**Katharine V. Smith, PhD, RN,** is associate professor emeritus at the University of Missouri Kansas City School of Nursing and Health Studies, Kanasas City, Missouri. Dr. Smith has received multiple grants, most of which have focused on aspects of teaching, advanced education, and nursing traineeships. Recent scholarship includes peer-viewed publications and national presentations on the use of simulation to teach legal and ethical content. She has also coauthored the textbook *Teaching Technologies in Nursing and the Health Professions* (2019). Dr. Smith has taught in both undergraduate and graduate nursing programs, facilitating advanced clinical projects through the early conceptual phases.

**Colleen Paramesh, DNP, APRN, NP-C,** collaborating author, is a clinical assistant professor and program director at the University of Kansas School of Nursing, Kansas City, Kansas. She teaches evidence-based practice and DNP project courses. Dr. Paramesh is a published author who has given multiple national presentations. She has received several teaching awards, including the Daisy Award for Extraordinary Faculty and the Phyllis Keeney Lawrence Teaching Award. In addition to her teaching responsibilities, Dr. Paramesh is a practicing nurse practitioner at The University of Kansas Health System.

# Proposal Writing for the DNP Project

**FOURTH EDITION**

Wanda Bonnel, PhD, APRN, ANEF

Katharine V. Smith, PhD, RN

Collaborating Author: Colleen Paramesh, DNP, APRN, NP-C

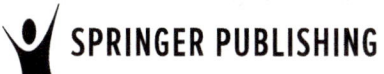

Copyright © 2026 Springer Publishing Company, LLC

All rights reserved.

First Springer Publishing edition 978-0-8261-2288-9 (2013); subsequent editions 2017, 2021

No part of this publication may be reproduced, stored in a retrieval system, or transmitted in any form or by any means, electronic, mechanical, photocopying, recording, or otherwise, without the prior permission of Springer Publishing Company, LLC, or authorization through payment of the appropriate fees to the Copyright Clearance Center, Inc., 222 Rosewood Drive, Danvers, MA 01923, 978-750-8400, fax 978-646-8600, info@copyright.com or at www.copyright.com.

Springer Publishing Company, LLC
902 Carnegie Center/Suite 140, Princeton, NJ 08540
www.springerpub.com
connect.springerpub.com

*Acquisitions Editor*: Joseph Morita
*Compositor*: Transforma
*Production Editor*: Diana Osborne

ISBN: 978-0-8261-7467-3
e-book ISBN: 978-0-8261-8829-8
DOI: 10.1891/9780826188298

**SUPPLEMENTS**:

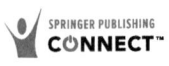 A robust set of instructor resources designed to supplement this text is located at http://connect.springerpub.com/content/book/978-0-8261-8829-8. Qualifying instructors may request access by emailing textbook@springerpub.com.

**Instructor Materials:**
*LMS Common Cartridge—All Instructor Resources ISBN*: 978-0-8261-0066-5
*Instructor Manual ISBN*: 978-0-8261-8864-9
*PowerPoint Slides ISBN*: 978-0-8261-5512-2
*Mapping to AACN Essentials ISBN*: 978-0-8261-6819-1
*Transition Guide to Fourth Edition ISBN*: 978-0-8261-7648-6

25 26 27 28 29 / 5 4 3 2 1

The author and the publisher of this Work have made every effort to use sources believed to be reliable to provide information that is accurate and compatible with the standards generally accepted at the time of publication. Because medical science is continually advancing, our knowledge base continues to expand. Therefore, as new information becomes available, changes in procedures become necessary. We recommend that the reader always consult current research and specific institutional policies before performing any clinical procedure or delivering any medication. The author and publisher shall not be liable for any special, consequential, or exemplary damages resulting, in whole or in part, from the readers' use of, or reliance on, the information contained in this book. The publisher has no responsibility for the persistence or accuracy of URLs for external or third-party Internet websites referred to in this publication and does not guarantee that any content on such websites is, or will remain, accurate or appropriate.

**Library of Congress Control Number: 2025000706**

Contact sales@springerpub.com to receive discount rates on bulk purchases.

***Publisher's Note:*** **New and used products purchased from third-party sellers are not guaranteed for quality, authenticity, or access to any included digital components.**

Printed in the United States of America.

# Contents

*Contributors of Proposal Abstracts and Project Examples*   vii
*Preface*   ix
*Acknowledgments*   xi
*Instructor Resources*   xiii

## Section I: Writing Your Proposal: Putting Your "Problem" in Context

1. Introduction: Why Write a Scholarly Proposal for the Clinical Project?   3
2. Using the Writing Plan as a Developmental Tool for the Advanced Clinical Project   11
3. Writing a Good Clinical Problem Statement and Gaining Project Context   19
4. Clinical Projects and Quality Improvement: Thinking "Big Picture"   27
5. Into the Literature: Gaining Best Evidence and Relevant Literature   35
6. Synthesizing Best Evidence and Literature Review   45
7. Framing the Advanced Clinical Project With Relevant Conceptual Frameworks   53

## Section II: Writing Your Proposal: Designing and Setting the Stage for Your Project

8. Addressing Outcomes Evaluation in the Advanced Clinical Project Proposal   63
9. Guiding the Advanced Clinical Project: The Purpose of a Purpose Statement   69
10. Mapping It Out: From Problem to Advanced Clinical Project Plan   77
11. Writing the Method Section: Organizing the Advanced Clinical Project Proposal   85
12. Gaining Credible Clinical Project Data: Being Systematic and Objective   95

## Section III: Writing Your Proposal: Adding the Detail for Proposal Completion

13. Writing the Data-Analysis Plans for Advanced Clinical Projects   103
14. Keeping Clinical Projects Ethical and Dependable   111
15. Finalizing the Proposal as a Professional Document: Reviewing, Editing, and Revising   117

## Section IV: Finalizing Your Proposal and Project: Next Steps

16. Moving the Proposal to Completed Project   127
17. Moving the Proposal to Written Final Report   135
18. Moving Your Completed Project to Dissemination and Further Scholarship   141

*Appendix A:*   Clinical Project Triangle   147
*Appendix B:*   Checklist for Planning or Self-Assessment of a Specific Project   149
*Appendix C:*   Proposal Abstract: "Improving the Care of Patients With Chronic Kidney Disease Using Evidence-Based Guidelines"   151
*Gwenyth Wagner*

*Appendix D:* Proposal Abstract: "Improving Diabetes Care Delivery in an Integrated Health Clinic" 153
*Jane Robinson*

*Appendix E:* Project Abstract: "Unit-Based Council Chairs' Perception of Unit-Based Councils" 155
*Sonya Curtis*

*Appendix F:* Proposal Abstract: "Descriptive Evidence Generating: Learning From Practitioner Owners of Clinics" 157
*Paula Israel*

*Appendix G:* Proposal Abstract: "Evidence Synthesis Plus: Anesthesia Considerations and Implications for Obese Pediatric Patients" 159
*Karri Arndt*

*Appendix H:* Proposal Abstract: "Evidence-Based Quality Improvement: Improving the Communication of Clinical Information Between Nurses and Physicians in Long-Term Care" 161
*Linda Kroeger*

*Index* 163

# Contributors of Proposal Abstracts and Project Examples

**Karri Arndt, DNP, APRN** Graduate, University of Kansas, Nurse Anesthesia Education, Kansas City, Kansas

**Sonya Curtis, DNP, MBA, RN, CNL** Graduate, University of Kansas School of Nursing, Kansas City, Kansas

**Paula Israel, DNP, APRN-BC** Graduate, University of Kansas School of Nursing, Kansas City, Kansas

**Linda Kroeger, DNP, APRN-FNP-BC** Graduate, University of Kansas School of Nursing, Kansas City, Kansas

**Roberta Mansfield, DNP, FNP-BC** Graduate, University of Kansas School of Nursing, Kansas City, Kansas

**Jane Robinson, DNP, FNP-BC** Graduate, University of Kansas School of Nursing, Kansas City, Kansas

**Gwenyth Wagner, DNP, APRN-C** Graduate, University of Kansas School of Nursing, Kansas City, Kansas

**Brigid Weyhofen, DNP, MSN, NEA-BC** Graduate, University of Kansas School of Nursing, Kansas City, Kansas

# Preface

Clinical projects provide opportunity to move from clinical challenges to problem-solving and competency in project development. At this unique time in history, diverse clinicians and student cohorts have the opportunity to enhance their skill sets in planning, writing, and implementing clinical project proposals. This text focuses on clinical application scholarship, the 2021 American Association of Colleges of Nursing (AACN) *Essentials* (2021), and student documentation of progress. The "must know" for gaining a set of clinical scholarship tools for writing a concise, scholarly project proposal are shared and students are guided through the necessary steps to project completion.

A well-written clinical project proposal is a form of scholarly communication and is expected in advanced practice. The text is broadly written to support diverse clinical project topics with a focus on quality improvement (QI). Although the uniqueness of advanced nursing practice allows no one proposal "formula," this text provides guides and templates for taking unique topics and relating these to common project models. Emphasis includes the use of the best evidence in projects with a focus on QI projects.

This book helps the reader to think prospectively about the big picture of the project, from start to finish, so important parts are not missed. This text guides the reader to integrate the project planning and proposal into DNP coursework. Information from courses such as theory, research, and statistics are used to develop a sound proposal for a quality advanced clinical project. A tool kit of resources, including the Project Triangle framework, guides graduate students and clinicians in attaining practical skills for proposal planning and writing. Using a reflective approach, guidelines, checklists and notebook documentation guides are provided to help clinicians and students develop quality clinical project proposals.

The following broad themes, corresponding to the main sections of the book, organize the 18 chapters in a logical flow toward completion of planning and writing a clinical project proposal, as well as implementing the project. Further scholarship and dissemination guides are provided. The unique chapter format reminds readers that development of a proposal is an integrative process, with many components that must be considered together.

1. **Writing Your Proposal: Putting Your "Problem" in Context**. Putting a clinical problem in context, including writing an introduction to the topic and problem statement, is important in making the case for a project. Context involves naming a specific setting and population as well as synthesizing the literature on a clinical topic and placing a project within that existing literature.

2. **Writing Your Proposal: Designing and Setting the Stage for Your Project**. The key points needed to create a scholarly method section that flows from a purpose statement are considered. Traditional QI tools and research methods are discussed as tools for DNP projects.

3. **Writing Your Proposal: Adding the Detail for Proposal Completion**. The importance of visualizing the finished product; editing for concise, clear language; and fine-tuning proposal methods and analyses are all considered.

4. **Finalizing Your Proposal and Project: Next Steps**. This section focuses on implementing specific quality-improvement projects and keeping clinical scholarship strong. Approaches to disseminating scholarly clinical projects are shared.

This book provides students with the tools necessary to implement their own scholarly practice. New to each chapter are QI Alerts serving as a reminder that each chapter has relevance to QI projects that are so important to enhanced clinical care. A Practice Scholarship Application reminder serves as a type of self-assessment for readers at chapter end for documenting accomplishments, review of the *Essentials*, and opportunity to complete competency documentation prompts for their project notebook. Online/Classroom Discussion prompts provide opportunity to apply content learned relevant to students proposal and project planning.

Key features used to engage readers continue from earlier editions; these include reflective questions, tips for making proposals complete and concise, exemplars, advice from DNP students and reader activities. This text helps develop reflective clinical scholars who can write about clinical challenges, propose solutions, and use the methods of QI and research to develop a tight scholarly project that can be shared with others.

*Wanda Bonnel*
*Katharine V. Smith*
*Colleen Paramesh*

## REFERENCE

American Association of Colleges of Nursing. (2021). *The essentials: Core competencies for professional nursing education.* https://www.aacnnursing.org/Portals/0/PDFs/Publications/Essentials-2021.pdf

# Acknowledgments

The authors acknowledge the many individuals who have influenced the writing of this book. We thank our students, who continue to help us learn; our university colleagues for sharing ongoing discussions and ideas; and program graduates, who have shared resources for chapter examples. Additionally, we thank our collaborating DNP author Colleen Paramesh. We thank our families for their ongoing encouragement and patience as we worked on this book. Thank you also to our Springer Publishing Company colleagues, especially Joseph Morita, for encouragement through the development of this fourth edition.

# Instructor Resources

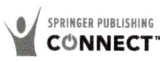 A robust set of instructor resources designed to supplement this text is located at http://connect.springerpub.com/content/book/978-0-8261-8829-8. Qualifying instructors may request access by emailing textbook@springerpub.com.

- LMS Common Cartridge—All Instructor Resources
- Instructor Manual—"Faculty Guide" includes the following assets for each chapter:
    - Student Learning Objectives
    - Chapter Overview
    - Faculty Questions and Teaching Tips
    - Retention Quiz for Students
- PowerPoint Slides
- Mapping to AACN *Essentials: Core Competencies for Professional Nursing Education*
- Transition Guide: Third Edition to Fourth Edition

# Proposal Writing for
the DNP Project

# SECTION I

## Writing Your Proposal: Putting Your "Problem" in Context

# 1. Introduction: Why Write a Scholarly Proposal for the Clinical Project?

## INITIAL THOUGHT

"What am I getting myself into?"

## CHAPTER CONTENT

- Reflective Questions
- Quality Improvement Alert
- Clinical Application Scholarship
- Clinical Application Scholarship and the American Association of Colleges of Nursing *Essentials*
- Proposal Writing for Scholarly Clinical Projects: Its Importance
- Writing a Clinical Project Proposal
- The Benefits of Reflection in Application Scholarship
- Making a Clinical Proposal Scholarly
- How Does the Reflective Clinician Use Evidence in Clinical Projects?
- Common Terms Related to Clinical Projects and Use of Best Evidence
- Clinical Scholarship: Seeking and Gaining a Mentor
- Introduction to the Clinical Project Triangle
- Beginning Project Checklist
- Advice From DNP Students
- Practice Scholarship Applications
- Summary and Key Points
- Websites for Further Review
- Next Chapter Up
- Online/Classroom Discussion
- Learning Activities
  - Beginning Writing Prompts
  - Checklist and Goal Setting: Readiness to Begin a Clinical Project

## REFLECTIVE QUESTIONS

As you begin your work on a clinical project proposal, there are benefits to reflecting on your goals. You have ideas for the clinical project and seek further thoughts to turn these ideas into scholarly proposals that will lead to tight, strong, and finished projects. The following reflective questions help you consider your writing plan and organize learning for this chapter. Which of the following do you have the most confidence responding to?

- What makes a project proposal important?
- What makes clinical application scholarship and the DNP project a good fit?
- How do project proposal competencies relate to the American Association of Colleges of Nursing (AACN) *Essentials* (2021)?
- What makes a clinical proposal scholarly?
- What are common terms related to best evidence and clinical project proposals?

Use the Practice Scholarship Applications (at the end of this chapter) to help document your learning from concept to competency, including the relevant American Association of Colleges of Nursing (AACN) *Essentials* (2021).

## QUALITY IMPROVEMENT ALERT

Many clinical projects use a quality improvement (QI) focus. This text describes broadly a variety of methods that have value in QI.

## CLINICAL APPLICATION SCHOLARSHIP

As you focus on clinical application scholarship, this text will help you prepare for and complete your DNP project. As you note in this textbook's table of contents, you will be moving chapter by chapter to sequence your learning experiences and progress from proposal development to project completion. This broad approach helps meet the need for diverse projects that meet the needs of diverse clinical populations and agencies.

The clinical project, a type of clinical application scholarship, is a product that shows you are accomplishing scholarly work and making a contribution to the professional community. As recognized by the AACN (2015), all DNP students should implement a project that demonstrates clinical scholarship. Boyer (1990) described not only the importance to the profession of sophisticated research programs, but also the value of clinical application scholarship. His classic framework for documenting scholarship includes frames of teaching, application, integration, and discovery.

The application construct, broadly considered as a clinical application focus, supports the value of DNP projects as scholarship. Quality-improvement (QI) projects, providing a good example of these products, provide opportunity to help others learn from your experiences and observations. To meet the definition of scholarship, components of product documentation, peer review, and publication or dissemination are required (Huber & Hutchings, 2005).

QI, an application scholarship and common clinical project approach, provides opportunity to move from ideas or concepts of interest to problem solving and competency in project development, as well as providing opportunity to demonstrate leadership in QI. These projects can also play a key role in documenting competency with select *Essentials*.

## CLINICAL APPLICATION SCHOLARSHIP AND THE AMERICAN ASSOCIATION OF COLLEGES OF NURSING *ESSENTIALS*

Why should you care about the *Essentials* and your DNP project as clinical application? To meet the changing needs of healthcare, AACN developed the 2021 educational *Essentials* to guide undergraduate and graduate student education (Giddens et al., 2022). The *Essentials* (AACN, 2021) describe key concepts relevant to the work of the nursing profession, and the contributions nursing graduates should be able to demonstrate. The AACN uses a competency-based approach in the *Essentials*, with competencies considered broad statements incorporating needed attitudes, knowledge, skills, and behaviors of learners (AACN, 2021). In some ways these serve as descriptors for the profession. The DNP project is considered an opportunity to apply and integrate DNP curriculum *Essentials* (Waldrop & Reynolds, 2023). Clinical projects lead to competency documentation in broad *Essentials* such as scholarship and science. Specific projects provide opportunity to show competency in other *Essentials* such as patient care and safety.

What do the *Essentials* mean to you? It's important to understand and make the *Essentials* about you as a nursing professional, to better understand what they are and why they exist. Demonstrating competency with select *Essentials*, via your DNP project, can also help identify learning gaps and show strengths, both for you and for your program. The *Essentials* can help you with the following (check off those that are important to you):

- being a professional by helping build the profession to ultimately enhance patient care
- helping identify your role/contribution to the profession
- helping document your outcomes/competencies by helping you document accountability
- showcasing your commitment and contributing to the profession

Related to application scholarship and the *Essentials* competencies, as you move through this text keeping a project notebook will provide opportunity to develop a personal summary and to document your project progress. As part of this notebook, you will complete reflective self-assessments to help consider your progress (and any further needed learning goals). At completion your project notebook will help you demonstrate your successful outcomes as well as readiness for leading future practice projects.

## PROPOSAL WRITING FOR SCHOLARLY CLINICAL PROJECTS: ITS IMPORTANCE

This book is designed to help you become a reflective clinical scholar and to write proposals for clinical projects that impact patient care. Clinical scholarship is key to advancing patient care and at this time of change in healthcare, advanced clinical nursing scholarship is needed more than ever. Although a DNP clinical project is designed to help improve patient care and safety for specific populations and systems, if carried out responsibly, strategies learned from a QI project may also lead to a broader professional contribution from which others might learn. Your role in becoming a clinical scholar continues to grow as you learn to write and implement proposals for clinical projects. As you plan a project that positively impacts your practice, writing a clinical project proposal is one aspect of that work.

## WRITING A CLINICAL PROJECT PROPOSAL

A proposal is a straightforward, logically organized, clear document that includes essential details that will guide a project. A proposal is considered the plan for how work will be designed to learn something important or improve a specific clinical problem. Proposals are further described as a presentation of ideas; a study justification; and a work plan, which serves as evidence of a chain of reasoning, project feasibility, and a binding contract for proposed work (Krathwohl & Smith, 2005). The term "project charter" is sometimes used to denote an abbreviated form of the proposal that focuses on the project action plan. The proposal plan needs to be logical, with the overall plan flowing from the problem and purpose statements. The proposal demonstrates how a need is met by this project and how it builds on previous work to address that need.

Leading and participating in scholarly clinical projects is one way you, as the advanced clinician, gain opportunities to make practice more visible to the public. Project aims or purposes can include promoting better patient care, supporting healthy people and community initiatives, and contributing to QI in healthcare systems. The specific purpose of your clinical project may relate to addressing patient care outcomes. As an advanced clinical practice nurse and leader, you develop clinical projects that integrate best evidence and consider contributions from other disciplines to improve clinical practice.

The proposal is a written portion of the scholarly clinical project that proposes what is to be done, and where, to complete that project. It also situates the project within the existing literature on the topic. Once the proposal for the clinical project is approved, the clinical project is ready to be implemented. Once the proposed activities are completed, the proposal document then is adapted to become the final project summary. To complete the final summary paper, after the project is completed, the proposal's Methods section is changed to past tense (to show completion), and new sections on project results and implications are added. Thus, this proposal is a useful, versatile document that

- serves as a form of communication or as a type of information sharing;
- proposes what is to be done (provides the plan or proposed project outline to be implemented) so others can understand, provide approval, or even replicate it;
- identifies important, related literature;
- provides information in a written and scholarly format through which others can quickly find key concepts;
- serves as a type of contract identifying clear expectations for a class or program requirement as well as the agency where the project will be completed; and
- serves as the basis for becoming a final project document that integrates the project proposal and outcomes.

This book guides you through steps that identify what you plan to do and helps you describe to others how you plan to do this. For example, the Institute of Medicine (2012) has identified the need for leadership in chronic-care management. Advanced practice nurses have the opportunity to address population health issues to improve public health. Approaches, such as education and QI, can be considered to help manage or control a chronic illness for a population subset. Designing a related clinical project could involve the following: naming a specific chronic illness and problem with a specific population and unit (such as osteoarthritis and pain management), selecting related concepts for further development or study that would lead to improved pain management (such as patient group coaching sessions on lifestyle modifications), reviewing the literature to determine the status of the evidence on the proposed concept, and framing this into a proposal for implementing or testing the best evidence to improve the care of patients with osteoarthritis pain.

## THE BENEFITS OF REFLECTION IN APPLICATION SCHOLARSHIP

Being an expert clinician or clinical leader comes with the responsibility of reflecting on practice issues to advance clinical patient care solutions. *Reflection* is a strategy that allows one to pause and think about what is going on; what is working or not working in a clinical or work-related situation. Reflection serves as a way to assess or identify gaps in clinical practice and move forward in clinical practice. Learning from these assessments often provides direction for future projects. As these ideas move to clinical project proposals, scholarly products and conversations that lead to clinical scholarship continue. As noted, you will be using reflective self-assessment as you complete components of your project notebook.

Critique of the current status of a particular care situation, for example, fall prevention, could involve addressing the problem from a systems perspective. This could incorporate reflection on the current unit or practice-site structures and processes (both needs and gaps) to gain positive outcomes. Listening, observing, and writing about this situation provide a starting point for related project development. In this situation, a reflective clinician asks: What is the team doing? How is it working? What could be better? These questions then lead to the identification of future clinical projects.

Scholarly writing is also related to reflection and scholarly dialogue; this scholarly dialogue involves reading the literature, communicating with others about that literature, and then developing the scholarly proposal. Further reflection and scholarly dialogue occur with completed project proposals, implementation of the projects, and finally sharing this scholarship via the literature. Scholarly writing of proposals includes using the methods of scholars and the language of the profession for disseminating the information contained in the clinical projects. Your project notebook provides a written communication summarizing the components of your project. It provides documentation or the basis for a tight scholarly project that can be shared with others.

## MAKING A CLINICAL PROPOSAL SCHOLARLY

Writing a scholarly proposal is part of a skill set needed to further clinical scholarship. Scholarly proposals provide a way to share, in a written and professional format, the important points of a major project. The proposal conveys not only what you will do, but why it is important that other people think about this topic. Your proposal then summarizes your plans; provides a road map for implementing plans; and delivers to others a plan that they can review, critique, and approve. Scholarly proposals, and then completed projects, provide a means to contribute to the body of knowledge and improve clinical practice.

While diverse approaches for completing a scholarly proposal exist, varying from a traditional scholarly proposal to an abbreviated charter or business prospectus, you will use the language of scholars and a commonly accepted format for organizing project proposals and final papers. This consistency in structure promotes ease of communication within nursing programs and the larger, interdisciplinary community. The common sections of a scholarly proposal are

- introduction with problem summary and purpose statement,

- literature review, and
- project methods.

Although clinical project topics are quite variable, in all cases some type of written proposal is a necessary component and serves as a project guide. In some ways completing a proposal is like putting together a puzzle and making sure all the pieces fit to give the best final picture. A scholarly proposal involves justifying and writing about your plan so that all of the clinical project pieces fit together.

A proposal serves as an important mechanism to clearly communicate about a proposed project. You will be communicating professionally, initially with your project team and later via professional presentations. Although this textbook lays out key proposal components chapter by chapter, it is important to consider the back-and-forth nature of each component; for example, further naming and detailing of the problem as a component of reviewing the literature. The art of scholarly proposing, in simple terms, includes

- starting with an important problem;
- situating that problem in the literature and identifying best evidence;
- framing the problem into a useful project, in writing, from which others can learn; and
- making the written project proposal scholarly and feasible.

## HOW DOES THE REFLECTIVE CLINICIAN USE EVIDENCE IN CLINICAL PROJECTS?

Scholarly dialogue includes reviewing best evidence in the literature as well as other professional sources of best evidence. Considering the state of the evidence can lead to further focus on the clinical problem. As you move forward in your proposal, you will begin asking questions that help you address how you will

- further understand your clinical problem/concept,
- gain a process for evidence-based practice,
- enhance quality care, and
- generate questions requiring further problem-solving and study.

Once you have a beginning understanding of what is available in the literature or best evidence, then you can make decisions on the type of project related to your problem/topic that is most needed. This allows you to focus broadly on using the evidence in advanced clinical projects such as the following:

- Synthesize the literature on topics to develop current best-practice summaries or protocols for testing; an example would be sharing a synthesis of best evidence and protocols for promoting the best anesthesia care for pediatric patients dealing with obesity.
- Contribute to the evidence by sharing new clinical data; an example would be surveying rural advanced practice nurses concerning their challenges and strategies for dealing with common rural population issues.
- Use and evaluate current best evidence protocols to implement QI projects with unique populations; an example would be teaching and evaluating the use of an evidence-based protocol on diabetes management in long-term care settings.

## COMMON TERMS RELATED TO CLINICAL PROJECTS AND USE OF BEST EVIDENCE

Many terms and models exist to describe the process of identifying best evidence for practice. Terms such as *translation of the evidence*, *research utilization*, and *evidence-based practice* can all relate to clinical projects and proposals. Although a commonality in these terms includes synthesizing the evidence, there are unique components to each, with basic descriptors that include the following:

- *Translation of the evidence*: Translate evidence into knowledge for practice and help staff become aware of and access evidence-based resources.
- *Research utilization*: Apply relevant studies to practice, after specific review and critique of each study.
- *Evidence-based practice*: Expand the concept of research utilization to include not only appropriate research in practice, but, when limited research evidence is available, incorporate other best evidence sources including opinions of expert clinicians; the patient preference for treatment is also a component.

Also, the concepts of evaluation, research, and QI are often discussed together. Again, there are similarities and differences in these basic terms, as well as frequent overlap of the concepts and methods used.

- *Evaluation*: Evaluative projects include systematic methods that judge the effectiveness of specific practices or policies.
- *Research*: Projects that involve systematic inquiry by using specified, disciplined methods of science in addressing problems or questions (Polit & Beck, 2020). Often research is equated with gaining new knowledge.
- *QI*: A framework, often based on systems theory, used to improve care. Such projects analyze a system's performance and search for ways to improve quality using a formal approach with systematic methods (Centers for Medicare & Medicaid Services [CMS], 2024).

Relevant to these concepts, evaluation is a broad project approach including methods used in both research and QI. Research studies typically build in more controls to be more generalizable to other settings and populations. QI is typically considered narrower in focus and for specific institutional use.

## CLINICAL SCHOLARSHIP: SEEKING AND GAINING A MENTOR

Seeking and gaining a mentor in the early stage of your work is an important and sometimes challenging task. Potential mentors should have expertise specific to the content, settings, and methods of an improved communication protocol. A mentor's availability, an interest in helping, and a strong commitment to your professional development are also important. The benefits of having a mentor are many, but, in particular, they include helping you avoid pitfalls in determining the feasibility or effectiveness of clinical project methods. When seeking a mentor, consider concepts of mutual readiness, opportunity, and resources available for support. For example, if your mentor is at a distance, what approaches will you use to facilitate conversations, and are both of you mutually interested in participating?

Finding a project mentor and using your project mentor(s) well are beneficial in all phases/aspects of project proposal development as well as during project implementation, evaluation, and completion. Consider the following strategies when seeking a mentor or to improve current work with a mentor:

- Focus on clear guidelines and expectations for both mentor and mentee.
- Establish regular meeting times whether via phone, face to face, or online.
- Find out when your mentor is available to read reports and what type of feedback your mentor is willing to give. Also, ask about the lead time required to review documents.
- Build a schedule for project reports or updates.
- Follow up on mentor's comments or suggestions.
- If your mentor is at a distance, discuss electronic communication strategies.

## INTRODUCTION TO THE CLINICAL PROJECT TRIANGLE

As you move forward with your clinical project, you should consider the benefits of using a clinical project triangle (Figure 1.1) and project checklist (Exhibit 1.1). The three points of the triangle include the project purpose, the methods, and the outcomes. This triangle helps hold the project together from a big-picture perspective and makes the project a cohesive whole. It is useful to begin a proposal with the triangle points in mind (subject to change as plans are finalized).

For example, in a sample QI communications project, the purpose was determining the outcomes of improved

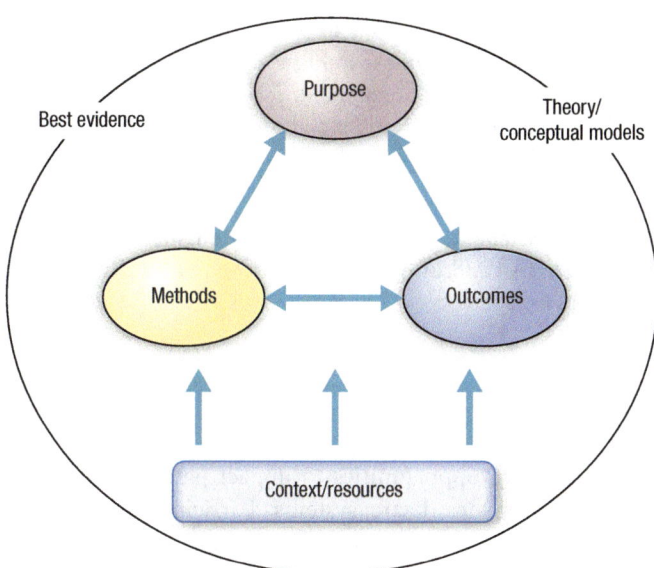

FIGURE 1.1 Clinical project triangle.

communication between nursing staff and providers in a long-term care setting. Methods were then selected that could help achieve the designated outcomes. The setting/context is named. As noted, the purpose is broad and the methods and outcomes will be more specific. The goal is for all project points on the triangle to mesh so that all aspects of the project are consistent and the overall project is coherent. Note the outer circle includes best evidence and theory/conceptual models that guide the central concepts.

## BEGINNING PROJECT CHECKLIST

Flowing from the project triangle is a beginning project checklist. Once you have identified a clinical problem and a tentative purpose statement, use the project checklist to consider tentative plans. As you move forward with your proposal, do a reflective review or critique of its strengths and weaknesses, and identify points you can strengthen. The project checklist in Exhibit 1.1 will assist you in this reflection.

Additionally, learn from the experience of DNP students who have preceded you in the proposal-writing process as given in the Advice From DNP Students box.

### PRACTICE SCHOLARSHIP APPLICATIONS

Consider your competency documentation plans. How will your project address select *Essentials*? Consider additions to your project notebook as you complete the following.

- *Concepts to competence*: In reviewing this chapter, think about your knowledge of proposal development. Review the Reflective Questions from the beginning of the chapter and self-assess on your progress with this chapter as you begin your work.

- *Essentials*: Review advanced level competencies and sub-competencies for the *Essentials* domains Knowledge for Nursing Practice, Scholarship for Nursing Practice, and Quality and Safety. Reflect on how they relate to your clinical project. How are these relevant to your planned DNP project and your professional career plans?
- *Project notebook*: Write and include a one-page written reflection that addresses your current or potential DNP project interests.

## SUMMARY AND KEY POINTS

Clinicians have opportunities to impact patient care in today's changing healthcare systems. Participating in application scholarship and being an expert clinician or clinical leader come with the responsibility of reflecting on practice issues and advancing clinical patient care solutions via scholarly projects. Clinical project proposals provide a way to begin naming the areas you would like to impact. Proposals for clinical projects directed at solving clinical problems can be implemented and shared as a form of scholarly practice. Points to recall from this chapter include the following:

- Consider the value of clinical application scholarship.
- Consider the importance of the *Essentials* in helping you name and describe scholarly outcomes and competencies.
- Recall the components of a scholarly proposal.
- Reap the benefits of reflection.
- Consider how best evidence affects your proposal.
- Be familiar with common terminology used in clinical projects.
- Secure a mentor and consider the clinical context for a project.
- Remember the clinical project triangle.

## WEBSITES FOR FURTHER REVIEW

Broad guides that provide background on DNP projects can be found on the websites of select national organizations. See the following examples:

- *Fact Sheet: The Doctor of Nursing Practice*:
  www.aacnnursing.org/Portals/0/PDFs/Facts-Sheets/DNP-Fact-Sheet.pdf
- *The Doctorate of Nursing Practice Nurse Practitioner Clinical Scholar*:
  https://cdn.ymaws.com/www.nonpf.org/resource/resmgr/docs/ClinicalScholarFINAL2016.pdf
- *Defining Scholarship for the Discipline of Nursing*:
  www.aacnnursing.org/news-information/position-statements-white-papers/defining-scholarship

### EXHIBIT 1.1 PROJECT CHECKLIST

As you begin your project proposal, use the following checklist to see if you are adequately considering each of the following. Indicate "agree" or "disagree" to confirm that each area has been thoroughly appraised. What are points you can strengthen?

| Concept | Have You Considered | Agree/Disagree |
|---|---|---|
| Evidence-based practice | What evidence is available to guide initiation and implementation of a particular project? | |
| Theory or conceptual model | What theory or model might best guide the project? | |
| Logistics/context with assessment of unit/setting | Have you assessed the need for your project and confirmed with clinical agency staff? | |
| | Have you assessed the feasibility of your project? | |
| | What are the facilitators/barriers for completing the project in a specific setting with a specific population? | |
| Purpose | Does the purpose flow from the identified problem? | |
| | What is to be achieved with the project? | |
| Methods | Have you considered diverse potential approaches to address your problem? | |
| | What is the best approach for your given problem and project purpose? | |
| Outcomes evaluation | What project outcomes are to be evaluated? | |
| | How will you know your project is successful? | |

## ADVICE FROM DNP STUDENTS

**Getting Started**

Stay with it.

- A project proposal needs to be a concise and clearly written paper containing information that is easily transferrable.
- It all seems foreign at first, but once you start working through it a little bit at a time and ask questions along the way, it starts to make sense.

Use the project triangle.

- This triangle helps you think through your project ideas and outline the work to be done.

**Tips for Getting Started**

As you begin your clinical project, here are some tips to help you:

- Schedule regular times to reflect on and write about a problem topic of interest for your project. Initially write from your personal experience and avoid getting bogged down in detail. Note any related facts, your reactions and feelings, as well as noting both frustrations and "aha" moments.
- Add something to your reflections at each scheduled work session. Even if you are not productive at first, this establishes the routine and sets the expectation to help you develop a regular work pattern.
- Prepare to address the questions your reflections raise: What evidence is available on this topic of interest? What is the state of current practice in a specified location or population? What value is there in further addressing this problem?

## NEXT CHAPTER UP

Chapter 2 provides a practical guide to getting started with your writing plan. The chapter offers ideas and tips on writing, asking the right questions, and making good choices to craft project proposals. Additionally plans for creating a project notebook are introduced.

## ONLINE/CLASSROOM DISCUSSION

In discussions with your colleagues, share responses to the following:

- What does it mean to be a clinical scholar? What examples can you provide?
- A professional has the responsibility to support the quality of practice (societal contract). Who is a role model for you? What can you learn from your role model related to clinical scholarship?
- How does practice scholarship add value to your healthcare organization?
- How will the project you are considering fit with select *Essentials*?

## LEARNING ACTIVITIES

### Beginning Writing Prompts

Writing prompts provide a way to reflect and get some ideas on paper. Use these prompts to brainstorm possibilities:

- Some of the big concerns or problems I see in my clinical work relate to …
- If there is one clinical or work-related problem I would fix, it would be … and the outcomes I would be interested in would include …
- The people and place factors that impact this problem are …
- If I could focus on just one aspect of this problem, it would be …

### Checklist and Goal Setting: Readiness to Begin a Clinical Project

On a scale of 1 (low) to 3 (high), how would you rate yourself on each of the following points? What further goals do you need to address?

At this point in time …

- I am motivated to help improve patient outcomes via advanced clinical projects.
- I have noted some beginning clinical challenges and have project ideas I would like to further develop.
- I am in a situation that supports moving forward with a clinical project.
- I am ready to communicate professionally via a written proposal.

## REFERENCES

American Association of Colleges of Nursing. (2015). *The doctor of nursing practice: Current issues and clarifying recommendations: Report from the Task Force on the implementaion of the DNP.* https://www.aacnnursing.org/Portals/42/DNP/DNP-Implementation.pdf

American Association of Colleges of Nursing. (2021). *The essentials: Core competencies for professional nursing education.* https://www.aacnnursing.org/Portals/0/PDFs/Publications/Essentials-2021.pdf

Boyer, E. L. (1990). *Scholarship reconsidered: Priorities of the professoriate.* Carnegie Foundation for the Advancement of Teaching.

Centers for Medicare & Medicaid Services. (2024). *Quality measurement and quality improvement.* https://www.cms.gov/medicare/quality-initiatives-patient-assessment-instruments/mms/quality-measure-and-quality-improvement-

Giddens, J., Douglas, J. P., & Conroy, S. (2022). The revised AACN essentials: Implications for nursing regulation. *Journal of Nursing Regulation, 12*(4), 16–22. https://doi.org/10.1016/S2155-8256(22)00009-6

Huber, M., & Hutchings, P. (2005). *The advancement of learning: Building the teaching commons*. Jossey-Bass.

Institute of Medicine. (2012). *Living well with chronic illness: A call for public health action*. National Academies Press.

Krathwohl, D., & Smith, N. (2005). *How to prepare a dissertation proposal: Suggestions for students in education and the social and behavioural sciences*. Syracuse University Press.

Polit, D., & Beck, C. T. (2020). *Nursing research: Generating and assessing evidence for nursing practice* (11th ed.). Lippincott Williams & Wilkins.

Waldrop, J., & Reynolds, S. (2023). Curricular revision to increase use of quality improvement principles in doctor of nursing practice projects. *The Journal for Nurse Practitioners, 19*(3), 104530. https://doi.org/10.1016/j.nurpra.2022.104530

# 2. Using the Writing Plan as a Developmental Tool for the Advanced Clinical Project

## INITIAL THOUGHT

"Good writing takes a lot of work."

## CHAPTER CONTENT

- Reflective Questions
- Quality Improvement Alert
- Considering Scholarly Writing and Reading Together
  - Writing as a Tool in Consider a Good Problem and Project Approach
  - Linking Scholarly Writing With Reading
- Self-Directed Writing: Prewriting and the Broad Writing Plan
  - Prewriting
  - Tips to Maintain Momentum for Your Writing Plan
- Drafting the Scholarly Writing Plan
- Strategies to Keep the Scholarly Writing Plan Moving Forward
  - Getting Started With Big-Picture Tools and Problem-Solving Strategies
  - Reflective-Writing Strategies
    - *The One-Page Early Reflection*
    - *Ongoing Reflective Journaling*
  - Tools to Help Document and Further the Writing Plan
    - *Decision Trails*
    - *Team Meetings*
  - Self-Editing
  - Peer and Mentor Reviews
- Advice From DNP Students
- Using the Project Notebook to Document Your Project Competencies
- Practice Scholarship Applications
- Summary and Key Points
- Websites for Further Review
- Next Chapter Up
- Online/Classroom Discussion
- Learning Activities
  - Writing Prompts
  - Checklist and Goal Setting for Generating a Writing Plan

## REFLECTIVE QUESTIONS

Clearly written communication is a powerful tool in healthcare. It is credited with avoiding system errors and promoting quality care. In Chapter 1, your focus was thinking about what you do as a clinician and beginning to identify where clinical improvements are needed as a project. You considered the importance of your scholarly project proposal. In this chapter, you begin to address the clear writing that is essential *to* the proposal; each section within the proposal has specific needs and guidelines that must be followed to comply with standards of scholarly writing. The following reflective questions organize learning for this chapter. With which of the following are you the most confident?

- Why is this writing plan important?
- What makes clinical scholarship and proposal writing go together?
- What does it mean to organize and draft a writing plan? Why focus on self-directed learning and writing?
- What strategies are used to begin and to keep the scholarly writing plan moving forward?
- What is the value of the project notebook to document your project process, products, and competencies?

Use the Practice Scholarship Applications (at the end of this chapter) to help document your learning from concept to competency, including the relevant American Association of Colleges of Nursing (AACN) *Essentials* (2021).

## QUALITY IMPROVEMENT ALERT

Good writing is good writing, whether for a class paper or a DNP quality improvement (QI) project. The project notebook serves as a tool to help you organize your DNP project.

A good clinical project, written first as a clinical proposal, guides and enhances project quality for credible outcomes. Reflective clinicians begin a proposal by seeing a problem, generating a plan for dealing with the problem through the proposal process, and then implementing the proposed clinical project. Reflective clinicians, as self-directed writers, follow steps that guide the proposal write-up, taking ideas and meshing them with project guidelines or templates to craft quality projects.

A written proposal is the first formal step of a clinical project and is a form of clinical scholarship. This chapter offers information about organizing and beginning the writing plan and as well discusses being a reflective clinician and sharing through writing. This chapter moves you forward in considering reading and writing together, gaining a plan for self-directed writing, drafting a scholarly writing plan, and strategies to use to keep the scholarly writing process moving along. The concept of developing a project notebook is introduced.

## CONSIDERING SCHOLARLY WRITING AND READING TOGETHER

### Writing as a Tool in Considering a Good Problem and Project Approach

The goal is to write a proposal that clearly names your project plans. This accomplishes three things: (a) it allows you to clarify what you will be doing in your project, (b) it helps others understand the intent of the project, and (c) it provides a map or guide so that others can understand the merit of the project and replicate the project in other settings. As you name and learn about specific clinical issues of interest, you will be reflecting and writing about them.

### Linking Scholarly Writing With Reading

At this stage of the clinical project, reading and writing fit together. While reading, you are gaining a big picture of the topic and planning how to situate your specific issue within its appropriate context (including both its setting and the available literature in the area).

- Use active reading to narrow the field (preview articles and consider questions to address further in reading).
- As you read, develop questions about studies and findings to address the who, what, where, and how outcomes are achieved.

Typically, you have focused on reading to learn more about specific practice concepts. At this point, you are also reading to consider approaches that might be used to help move your clinical project forward. What do you learn from what others have done that can be used to package projects in meaningful ways to benefit colleagues, staff, and students?

## SELF-DIRECTED WRITING: PREWRITING AND THE BROAD WRITING PLAN

Why should you care about the writing plan? Because your hours are limited, you have to maximize your use of those hours. The writing plan is important because it helps outline the important points that need to be addressed in developing your proposal. Just as quality improvement and planning in nursing is central to patient care, the larger clinical project can use a similar "care plan" approach in assessing project need, clearly stating the problem, outlining possible approaches, and then selecting the best approach for the situation. Documenting how the project outcomes will be evaluated is also included.

### Prewriting

Prewriting occurs before official proposal writing starts. This refers to the point at which you get organized and ready to write. It can include getting yourself to your writing place; sticking to the time you have allotted; having a beverage in hand; and getting sufficient reading, thinking, and exploring done to lead your writing down the best path (putting together reading notes that can later be cited is also useful).

Prewriting also provides an opportunity for early organization of thoughts or to clarify problems, as well as to help identify what your project is *not* about (Wolcott, 2008). Because this prewriting helps focus your ideas, the project becomes more reasonable and then becomes more doable. Your actual problem can become clearer through this process and provide opportunities to consider other phases of the work.

Sometimes reflecting on broad questions serves as a good prewriting tool. For example, why is this topic interesting to me? Specific writing tools, such as project reflective journals, help you document your work; the acts of reflecting and journaling help assess what is working or not with your project plans. Getting-started tips for organizing a writing plan, including your writing time and space, include the following:

- *When to write?* When thinking about your time organization, does your plan include a calendar and a clock? Are you a morning or night person? What's compatible with your personal and family life?
- *Where to write?* Your writing space counts, too. Do you require a quiet, peaceful place to write or can you write anywhere? Often selecting one central writing area, with organized supplies and resources, helps writing efficiency. An added bonus is finding a spot where you can spread out and not have to pick up every time after you have finished working.
- *What to write?* Anything; just start to get something on paper. Then work your way into the specific proposal components you are addressing.

### Tips to Maintain Momentum for Your Writing Plan

Many life events will distract you from writing. Try to put writing first for selected time periods (other than emergencies). Tips for keeping momentum include the following:

- Develop a big-picture project map that helps you stay on track.
- Be realistic in setting goals or when making doable plans; describe deliverables.

- Organize tasks by creating a timeline and check it regularly.
- Be clear and enthusiastic about goals.
- Identify a mentor or colleague as a support person.
- Identify someone besides yourself to whom you're responsible for accomplishing specified work and achieving due dates.

## DRAFTING THE SCHOLARLY WRITING PLAN

Organization is important and is different for scholarly proposals (or a project charter) than it is for other types of writing. Although textbooks are written for broad audiences to highlight and summarize key content areas, in a clinical proposal the format becomes more prescriptive. For example, at least three focused sections are typically addressed in scholarly proposals, including (a) the introduction (with problem summary and project purpose statement), (b) literature review and synthesis, and (c) methods. Specific sections, such as the Methods subsection, then address further project components (project design, any evidence-based implementation plans, sample, data collection, and data-analysis plans). Future chapters elaborate on these topics.

To begin organizing the scholarly writing plan, reflective questions and written responses can help make the connections to puzzling problems. Sample questions include the following:

- *What will you be doing?* When writing the scholarly proposal, there are multiple concepts to consider. This includes addressing what is known about your problem or clinical project topic and including the literature review (what others have written on the subject). You will also explain the plan for your project.
- *Who will you be writing for?* There are different rules/guidelines for different audiences. Are you writing for a hospital clinical project committee? A research review board? A faculty member? Who else are you writing this proposal for? Spend time considering your various audiences and the implications of these different groups for the project proposal expectations and requirements.
- *What tools/techniques are available?* It's important to know about the available resources for increasing efficiency as well as effectiveness. In addition to the broad proposal guidelines outlined in this text, often specific guidelines are available to assist you in crafting clinical project proposals, with specific purposes such as coursework or grant funding. To begin, what specific guidelines are available to guide you in crafting the proposal? Are there templates to guide completion? Is there a time frame for proposal completion? Is there a page limit? From a practical perspective, drafting an early table of contents that outlines all the required components is a useful strategy.
- *What are your qualifications?* What education and experiences have prepared you to propose and write a specific project proposal? Or to use specific methods? Or even study the proposed concept? Just as an athlete would not undertake a major athletic event without preparing, it is important that you also have or gain the background, education, and skills needed to propose and complete the clinical project.
- *Are there practical concerns or ethical issues involved in a particular topic?* As part of clinical projects, both practical and ethical issues and concerns must be addressed. For example, if you would like to learn more about patient function in specific home settings for your elderly population, what practical issues must be addressed in making home visits? What potential ethical issues might need to be addressed if you wanted to take videos of the patient in the home for analysis?
- *Will you be able to carry out the project you are proposing?* Striving for a project that is not too big and not too small can be a challenge when you first begin your project planning. Mentor and peer review can provide the benefit of additional perspectives to help deal with finding the proper balance.

## STRATEGIES TO KEEP THE SCHOLARLY WRITING PLAN MOVING FORWARD

Motivation for pursuing clinical projects is often high while thinking and planning, but students anecdotally share that actually writing the proposal can be a challenge. Considering the proposal's "big picture" and keeping the end result in mind can be a form of motivation. Writing the proposal with the project triangle in mind, with the goal of ultimately getting the purpose, methods, and outcomes in alignment, provides the foundation for a well-organized clinical project that helps improve clinical practice.

### Getting Started With Big-Picture Tools and Problem-Solving Strategies

All scholarly writers need a good starting point and tools to keep moving their writing forward. Starting with a good clinical problem (Chapter 3) can help motivate you and keep you going. For example, finding an area of interest or a concern/challenge (that you believe will truly improve patient care) and then studying it, making a quick assessment of related concepts and issues, can be helpful.

*Concept-mapping tools*, for example, provide a visual approach to help name your problem and its context. Developing concept maps provides a beginning reflective activity. Maps help you think about key points surrounding a particular problem and provide potential options to consider before making your case as to why this is an important problem. They have the benefit of helping visualize multiple related concepts or issues that may be tangential to or influence the problem.

*Problem-solving* fits with concept mapping as a brainstorming tool to identify possible antecedents to the problem and to identify particular patterns that emerge. First, visualize or push your thinking to the big picture of the problem to better understand it before moving on to the full project. Other tools used to visualize big-picture issues include outlining and diagramming approaches. These have the benefit of exposing the big picture of potential aggravating or causative factors.

*Outlining* is described as an art and offers the following benefits: Firms up thinking, organizes materials, and yields a logical step-by-step method. Providing a type of visual impression, an outline can help identify gaps or excesses in writing plans, promoting unity and emphasis on key points (Savers, 2017). Some use a broad outline format, focusing only on broad concepts as a guide, rather than focusing on the details. Experiment with both and see which is more helpful to you.

*Using a fishbone-type diagram* can help identify important factors or components that influence problems. Similar to concept maps, these arrow-type diagrams help organize thinking on specific topics. The fishbone diagram provides direction in naming potential challenges affecting one problem area. Using a systems perspective, planning arrows remind you to consider structure-and-process issues that may be impacting particular topics and outcomes. Moving beyond basic concept identification, further diagramming can help identify possible interrelations (such as spider diagrams or extended Venn diagrams). Asking who, what, when, and where can also help diagram the topic/plan.

*Problem-solving question prompts* can help you to brainstorm. Brainstorming, or rapidly generating ideas relevant to your topic, is valuable as you begin a project. This includes asking the right questions such as: What if? and I wonder whether…?

## Reflective-Writing Strategies

Reflection provides an opportunity to make sense of experiences and can lead to quality-improvement opportunities (Kaplan et al., 2013; Sherwood & Horton-Deutsch, 2017). Reflection is a key tool to use not only to begin writing, but also to keep progressing. Reflection (along with scholarly dialogue and reflective writing) is a tool that can also help evaluate clinical challenges, generate further questions, and potentially lead to problem solutions. Reflective responses to questions can help focus and stimulate thinking, encouraging new thoughts and responses to challenges.

### The One-Page Early Reflection

One approach to using reflection as you begin a project is to start by writing about why you chose a particular topic. This would include, for example, the interests that led you to this topic including the identified need from your clinical agency.

If you have several topics in mind, complete a one-page reflective paper on each topic that addresses the following: What do I already know/think/feel about this topic? What questions do I still have? These reflections help address why these topics/projects are important and interesting to you and the clinical value they will provide to you and your clinical agency. Other reflective-writing techniques can be helpful at various points in the project.

### Ongoing Reflective Journaling

Ongoing journaling, spending even 10 to 15 minutes a day writing about a project, can support ongoing progress and project success. It is important to establish the writing routine or habit and get something related to the project on paper. For a jump start, combine this habit with already established rituals, such as a morning cup of coffee.

- *Answering structured questions or using writing prompts* to guide written reflections adds more direction to journaling. This practice promotes tracking what you already know about your project and helps identify areas needing further attention or further inquiry (Wolcott, 2008). Consider using the reflective questions incorporated throughout this text as writing prompts to get you going and keep you going.

- *Free writing* leads to learning more about your thoughts and subsequently organizing those thoughts. Free writing involves letting words flow without concern for spelling, edits, or others' eyes. The goal is to simply get content/thoughts on paper. You then have something to edit and share with colleagues that conveys your thoughts for further discussion.

## Tools to Help Document and Further the Writing Plan

Especially when working on a large project over time, there are benefits to outlining and using record-keeping tools that help track factual information, resources, and project decisions.

### Decision Trails

Sometimes called audit trails, decision trails are factual records of decisions made. They include keeping an annotated list of your work and decisions as you go along. This provides a record of what actually has been done and also helps you remember why you made the decisions you did, serving as a type of summary. It allows you to keep track of processes undertaken and ongoing challenges as well as accomplishments. The value of decision trails includes providing a reflective reminder of project choices.

As noted by one DNP student: "My decision trail, or paper trail, has been more than beneficial. It helps to identify where

I have been and my trajectory along the path toward my accomplishments. It has prevented me from redoing a task or revisiting a problem."

### Team Meetings

Meeting with team members as your project progresses is additionally needed. It is important to maintain clear dialogue with team members, as well as written follow-up communication. When meeting and communicating with your project mentor or other team members, have an agenda prepared. This includes a list of specific questions you would like to discuss. Listen actively to gain the other person's viewpoint.

Send follow-up communication to confirm clear and consistent understanding on both parts. Share, for example, "This is what I heard at our meeting and these are the points I will follow-up on." When you are asked to make revisions, make sure you show on your follow-up document where those changes were made (e.g., using different text colors or the track changes feature in Microsoft Word).

### Self-Editing

Begin to self-edit, a process in which you read and reread your written work to make sure it clearly states your intended ideas. As the number of times you read your own words increases, it is easy to start gliding over them too quickly to edit effectively, so it is helpful to read your work aloud to slow yourself down and to hear different inflections that can be read into your wording and punctuation choices. It is particularly useful to evaluate your work against an available proposal rubric. This step often helps one avoid missing important proposal components. Also, putting the paper aside and then revisiting it after several days provides an opportunity for clearer self-evaluation of the writing.

### Peer and Mentor Reviews

Peer and mentor reviews provide good approaches to editing. Peer review includes reviewing, interpreting, and communicating evaluative information to or from a colleague. This can be a formal or informal process that helps nurses provide feedback to peers based on specific criteria. Typically, this is an interactive process and involves the use of specified guidelines or rubrics based on criteria to guide the feedback. Remember that a combination of positive and constructive feedback is most helpful—while exclusively positive feedback might feel good and exclusively negative feedback seem unhelpful, neither alone makes a good critique; be sure to provide a balance of positive and constructive comments.

Seeking formal reviews from mentors is also key. Points to consider include the following:

- Be proactive in seeking/gaining feedback on your writing trouble spots.

- If you note trouble spots in your writing, rework what you have written. If you cannot give up any of your initial paragraph drafts, open a file named "extra" to copy and paste information for potential future use.

- Seek out writing centers at schools or from private resources to guide you if you are experiencing problems conveying your thoughts clearly. Writing centers provide guidance, not on your content, but on your process for organizing and conveying written information.

Also, learn from the experience of DNP students who have preceded you in the proposal-writing process. Their advice is presented in the following.

---

**ADVICE FROM DNP STUDENTS**

**Beginning to Write Your Proposal**

Make sure you know the proposal guidelines.

- Clearly identify expectations and additional resources to assist you in proposal development.

Think about your proposal in sections (similar to scholarly articles).

- Try to go step by step. The various steps need to be considered in a systematic way to organize and develop a successful project.
- It helps to know how to "talk the research language."

Use an outline to help you know ahead of time what you will be writing.

- Think about the process (or parts/sections) for pulling together the parts of a DNP proposal.
- Clearly outline the method subsection. It is extremely helpful to do the outline first. This facilitates writing.

Focus on reflection.

- It helps to constantly reflect on where you are in your project proposal. When you get stuck, go back to the project questions and reflect; it helps.

**Tips for Getting Started**

As you begin your writing, here are some tips to help you:

- Stay focused on the project topic.
- Get something written down.
- Address the beginning/middle/end formula, as you would in speech class, to help you outline a section of the proposal. In addition to the main "middle" message, the Introduction summarizes what you tell the reader and why it is important. An effective conclusion then summarizes what has been accomplished.
- Use time-management strategies, such as scheduling time on your calendar, for clinical proposal writing.
- Remember your decision trail and keep journaling to record your ideas/decisions.

## USING THE PROJECT NOTEBOOK TO DOCUMENT YOUR PROJECT COMPETENCIES

Project notebooks are useful tools in documenting scholarship and competency. For purposes of this text, a project notebook will be considered a purposeful collection of products that documents your efforts, progress, and achievement in your DNP clinical project. It includes your reflections on your work and progress. A reflective component allows you to self-assess on your work and identify both strengths and weaknesses as well as ongoing needs of the project. It can serve as a type of debriefing.

Reflections can also help identify how your project fits or relates to the *Essentials*. Naming and sharing your project via this project notebook shows how outcomes will be gained. It helps avoid the concept of a "black box" (where others are left to wonder how and why the project pieces and outcomes came together).

Even if a brief proposal format, such as a proposal charter, rather than a longer scholarly document is supported by your DNP program, the project notebook assists you personally to keep track of your process and show your personal outcomes. The project notebook provides a record of your work, your project choices and rationales, and serves as a type of decision trail. Because projects consist of both process and products, the project notebook can serve as the primary location to post ongoing progress and product documents during a semester and beyond. The project notebook helps avoid a random or mixed stack of papers from components of your project work spread across your desk or computer. Consider the project notebook's value for your work:

- It describes the approaches to specific proposal activities by naming and showing what you have done and why this matters.
- It describes and documents your project components, moving from concept to competency in documenting the *Essentials*.
- It allows reflection on your process and products as self-assessment, a component of professional development.
- It summarizes what has been accomplished (and how) and provides potential that others could replicate for a similar project in their own settings. It could even set the stage for your own goal setting, helping determine what's next.

Here are some tips to set up your project notebook, as you begin your work:

- Create your empty notebook (electronic or hard copy).
- Use a good table of contents (it's a guide for you and your readers).
- As you create your table of contents use the beginning/middle/end consideration for divider headings (the introductory summary, the middle details of the project, and the endings as to what has been accomplished). You may want to work backward from your final project idea to identify what needed pieces might be done as miniprojects during your clinical practicum.
- Consider your concepts to competency plans. What are you learning and how will you show this?
- Include reflection on each component. Why is each outcome document or process summary important to your project? To your clients or populations or staff? To the profession?
- The reflective summary section can also address questions such as what were your challenges and strengths in developing this product?

### PRACTICE SCHOLARSHIP APPLICATIONS

Consider your competency documentation plans. How will your project address select *Essentials*? Consider additions to your project notebook as you complete the following.

- *Concepts to competence*: After reviewing this chapter, evaluate your scholarly writing needs. What is your self-assessment of your writing abilities? What plan can help you gain competencies in developing your project? How can a reflective project notebook contribute?
- *Essentials*: How are the domains Knowledge for Nursing Practice and Scholarship for Nursing Practice relevant to your planned DNP project and your professional career plans? Review advanced level competencies and subcompetencies for each of these *Essentials* domains and reflect on how they relate to your clinical project.
- *Project notebook*: Complete a written reflection on your own quality improvement efforts. What writing plan have you developed to start your project proposal? Consider or self-assess your progress in gaining a quality improvement perspective on your writing.

## SUMMARY AND KEY POINTS

Although much of this chapter focused on approaches to writing a clinical project proposal, it was also about tools that make writing a part of clinical scholarship. Writing is a way to name and package what you are doing or planning to do. A writing plan can lead to successful proposals that then lead to successful clinical projects. The self-directed writer becomes adept at organizing time, place, and space. There are various tools to help the clinician writer stay motivated and organized to move forward with writing tasks for clinical projects. Key points to recall from this chapter include the following:

- Link scholarly writing with active reading and questioning.
- Use writing as a tool in considering a good problem and project approaches. Begin by asking questions such as who am I writing for and what are the guidelines.

- Draft an early version of the project plan by addressing practical questions such as who, what, and is this doable.
- Prewrite and maintain momentum with an organized plan, including when and where to write.
- Keep the scholarly writing plan moving forward using tools such as concept mapping, planning arrows, reflective writing, early written reflections, and ongoing reflective journaling.
- Schedule communications with the project team, including your mentor, and seek periodic writing reviews.
- Learn the skills of self-editing and peer review to help move your proposal forward.
- Use the project notebook to document your project process, products, and project competencies.

## WEBSITES FOR FURTHER REVIEW

Diverse writing and communication resources exist. Useful resources as you begin your project include the following:

- *Communication Skills* (a toolkit for effective communication skills from MindTools):
  www.mindtools.com/pages/main/communication_skills.htm
- *How to Improve Writing Skills in English as a Second Language* (in addition to graduate program writing centers, consider using select web resources for tips on challenges):
  https://linguisity.com/posts/how-to-improve-writing-skills-in-english-as-a-second-language-a-comprehensive-guide
- *National Standards for Culturally and Linguistically Appropriate Services in Health and Health Care* (when working with patient populations with select challenges, consider resources for tips on challenges):
  https://thinkculturalhealth.hhs.gov/clas

## NEXT CHAPTER UP

How do you shape the problem statement? You have ideas and a plan for writing; now it is time to focus on organizing information on one specific problem area. Moving from the messy "problem" to the real issue and fine-tuning the problem statement is the next step.

### ONLINE/CLASSROOM DISCUSSION

- What are your personal scholarly writing experiences? What tips can you share with student colleagues on how you organize your writing plan? What strategies do you use to begin and to keep your writing plan moving forward?

## LEARNING ACTIVITIES

### Writing Prompts

Writing prompts provide a way to reflect and get some ideas written down. Use these prompts to brainstorm possibilities.

- I want to work more with this topic because…
- My background will help in the following ways…
- Areas in which I still need to gain knowledge/skill include…
- A beginning plan for gaining these skills includes…

### Checklist and Goal Setting for Generating a Writing Plan

To which of the following can you add a checkmark? Which of the following need to be further addressed?

Are you…

- writing regularly with reasonable ease?
- focusing fully on what you are to be writing?
- avoiding distractions to your reading and writing?
- using peers/advisors when needed?
- using an efficient writing process?
- moving forward?

Do you…

- have a project proposal writing timetable?
- feel good about your writing process?
- have a process that's working for you?
- have a steady writing pace that feels reasonable?
- have a pace consistent with your calendar for finishing the project proposal?
- have your project notebook started?

## REFERENCES

Kaplan, M., Silver, N., LaVaque-Manty, D., & Meizlish, D. (2013). *Using reflection and metacognition to improve student learning: Across the disciplines, across the academy*. Stylus Publishing.

Savers, C. (2017). *Anatomy of writing for publication for nurses* (3rd ed.). Sigma Theta Tau International.

Sherwood, G., & Horton-Deutsch, S. (2017). *Reflective practice: Transforming education and improving outcomes* (2nd ed.). Sigma Theta Tau International.

Wolcott, H. (2008). *Writing up qualitative research*. Sage Publication.

# 3. Writing a Good Clinical Problem Statement and Gaining Project Context

## INITIAL THOUGHT

"Problems, problems; there are so many clinical problems!"

## CHAPTER CONTENT

- Reflective Questions
- Quality Improvement Alert
- From Area of Concern to Problem Statement
  - Where Do Areas of Concern or Problems Come From?
- Clinical Settings and Clinical Practicum Mentors
- Focusing Your Area of Concern: The What and the Where
- Focusing the Problem
  - Bringing Ideas Into Shape
  - Narrowing the Topic
  - Clarifying the Problem Name and Description
  - Describing Context and Setting Boundaries
- What Makes This a Good and Important Problem to Study?
- Introducing the Problem in the Proposal
  - Problem Significance
  - Fine-Tuning the Problem Statement
  - Common Challenges With Problem Statements
  - Peer Review of Problem Statements
  - Using the Title to Help Convey the Project Intent
  - Project Triangle
- Advice From DNP Students
- Practice Scholarship Applications
- Summary and Key Points
- Websites for Further Review
- Next Chapter Up
- Online/Classroom Discussion
- Learning Activities
  - For Your Project Notebook: Your Story Related to Your Topic of Interest
  - Further Reflective-Writing Prompts
  - To-Do List
  - Readiness to Proceed

## REFLECTIVE QUESTIONS

In Chapter 2, you learned about tips for organizing your writing. In this chapter, the focus is on determining and naming the problem that is the subject of your writing, putting that problem in context, and creating a written problem statement. The following reflective questions organize learning for this chapter. With which of the following are you the most confident:

- Which areas of clinical practice do you find most interesting or problematic?
- What problematic areas of clinical practice, if changed, could improve patient care?
- Can you put these problematic areas in context of your clinical setting?
- Are you able to clarify the problem names and their descriptions/definitions?
- Can you explain the significance of finding a solution to the problems?

Use the Practice Scholarship Applications (at the end of this chapter) to help document your learning from concept to competency, including the relevant American Association of Colleges of Nursing (AACN) *Essentials* (2021).

### QUALITY IMPROVEMENT ALERT

Clearly naming an important clinical problem is a key component of quality improvement (QI). What problem will you work on to help improve an organizational or population concern?

## FROM AREA OF CONCERN TO PROBLEM STATEMENT

This chapter is about taking an area of concern and turning it into a clearly named problem. Broadly described, a problem refers to a situation that needs a solution. A clinical problem relates to situations or topics that provide clinicians and clinical leaders opportunities to improve patient care and can lead to evaluating and packaging new approaches that promote safe care delivery and products for clinical education and leadership. Good problems for projects have good practical implications, are well delineated, and promote personal and career interests (Krathwohl & Smith, 2005). The final problem statement sets the stage for generating the project purpose and methods for completing the work.

## Where Do Areas of Concern or Problems Come From?

As you know, clinical problems come in all shapes and sizes. As a good reflective clinician, you probably have many "problem" ideas already. It is important to look around and see what current challenges exist in your clinical setting. What is happening, or not happening, that impacts safe, quality care? Current nursing specialty problems or issues that may also serve as project ideas are often described via professional nursing meetings, funding sources, and specialty newsletters.

Clinical problems can be unique or common. Some are relevant to specific areas of a unique practice setting. Others might be relevant to diverse settings or broad health-promotion issues of populations. Sample brainstorming options to help you generate specific clinical problem areas include the following:

- Are you wondering about, or have you uncovered any clinical unit problems from recent practice experiences? Are you considering QI needs? Could there be a better way of doing things related to this concern?
- Are you thinking about ways to improve staff education on clinical topics, documentation standards, or interprofessional practices on clinical topics? For example, are there appropriate pain-management protocols for those with late stage dementia?
- Are you having conversations with others about reviewing competence in clinical practice settings? Are staff demonstrating current clinical competencies that match current national standards? What practice concerns do your colleagues identify?

## CLINICAL SETTINGS AND CLINICAL PRACTICUM MENTORS

Clinical practicum work and clinical mentors can provide important connections to potential clinical projects and application scholarship. As you work with mentors within your practicum you have opportunity to gain needed project ideas.

In this chapter, as part of thinking about a problem or concern that you want to focus on for your clinical project, several "problem" aspects are considered. For example, how do you focus a problem for study? How do you know it is an important problem that needs to be addressed in your clinical work or practicum settings? How do you know that you are choosing a feasible problem to pursue as a scholarly clinical project?

## FOCUSING YOUR AREA OF CONCERN: THE WHAT AND THE WHERE

Where will you plan to identify a clinical problem and complete your project? Clinical work or practicum settings might provide valuable opportunities for problem identification as well as opportunity to document the concern of interest. Seeking input from clinical partners will be central to your work.

While different graduate programs have different approaches to the clinical practicum, the practicum setting often provides opportunities that could involve project pieces such as identifying and describing a specific problem. Opportunities can exist as you work with your preceptor or mentor and other unit/agency clinical stakeholders to identity and describe problems of concern as well as helping you make the case for your project. Thinking further about this, if, for example, you are in a leadership or direct care practicum:

- Can you use your practicum as opportunity to identify needs from different perspectives? For example, what does the program/unit director worry about? What concerns do you see patients having? Reflecting as a graduate student, what problems do you note? Are there similar themes in these diverse concerns? Do some ideas have more priority than others?
- Can you gain more information on your area of concern by reviewing unit policies, attending meetings and workshops, or interviewing staff? What are common agenda items or concerns that you are hearing?
- When in a direct patient care role, can you complete project components during this time (e.g., documenting project need with data from unit electronic records or your own clinical logs)? If you are working with a specific population (in the community or clinical agency), can you gain "needs" data from select agency records, online reports, or other sources?

As you follow up on these project opportunities, can you gain data to help document specific needs related to your problem of concern, perhaps using your practicum to include sequential project pieces? This might include completing mini projects (or practicum deliverables); setting up, for example, a patient needs assessment one semester, and a specific organizational assessment another.

Considering these possibilities you might, for example, identify a problem such as lack of good diabetes follow-up care in a rural clinical setting. Part of your practice work might include documenting the need for a rural diabetes clinic (generating patient data from electronic resources and listening to patient concerns; generating clinical agency needs from resource reviews such patient education materials; reviewing provider screening forms and other organizational resources such as the American Diabetes Association Standards). Over the course of the practicum, these approaches can help describe and narrow the problem as well as gaining important needs assessment data, even setting the stage for your project and engaging your practice partners.

## FOCUSING THE PROBLEM

### Bringing Ideas into Shape

Once you have an idea or topic of concern, the goal is to take this broad problem area and turn it first into a focused problem and then a specific problem statement, moving from a general problem to a specific problem. Areas of concern are different from focused problems as they typically involve numerous broad interacting issues rather than a detailed focused problem. For example, as a clinical leader in long-term care, describing the group dining setting for frail elders as a "mess" may accurately state an area of concern, but it lacks direction for improving the elders' dining situation. Moving from a broad, fuzzy area of concern to a specific problem(s) is one of the first parts of project development. What do you specifically mean by your "problem?" In this group dining situation, are there staffing issues? A lack of adaptive equipment? Poor environmental arrangements?

When you have identified a broad area of concern, consider whether any of the additional brainstorming tools could be used to further focus the problem. Brainstorming tools can help not only first identify big-picture issues (e.g., the top of a funnel) but also in narrowing down to a more specific aspect of a broad problem. These tools can also help clearly identify what the problem or issue is and what the surrounding factors are. Additional strategies to use to help clarify the problem and to consider a problem's context (which are reviewed further in Chapter 4) include

- root cause analyses or fishbone diagrams, which help name and organize the potential factors that can be impacting a problem;
- concept maps or concentric-circle diagrams; and
- addressing the who, what, why, where, and when related to a particular problem, which can also help focus a problem.

Again, early project work involves making sure you are identifying and naming a problem that can be focused. Once the problem is named, you will go on to write a problem statement and then, following that, you will write the project purpose statement. Concurrent with this writing process, you will be searching the literature. The literature review determines what is already known and not known about this clinical problem in the profession. It addresses whether and/or how others have considered or addressed this or similar problems.

The literature related to your area of concern not only helps with naming and describing the problem of interest but can also help as you move forward in thinking about a potential project plan. The literature review helps you identify whether there are numerous scholarly publications on the topic, suggesting that your problem topic is evidence rich, or conversely, that there are few publications offering limited evidence related to your topic. It addresses whether the evidence you are finding can help with further solution planning. For example, as you have conversations with other professionals about the group dining room in your long-term care setting, your use of problem-solving models and review of the literature can help identify various issues that lead to problems within this setting.

Sample approaches used to gain ideas on topics of interest or problem areas include

- reading broadly and then becoming more specialized,
- reviewing tables of contents for sample naming of problems or approaches to a problem,
- reviewing textbooks on a topic of interest to identify broad challenges,
- seeking synthesis articles first and then following up with specific studies, and
- contacting experts in the field.

### Narrowing the Topic

Once you begin describing the problem, there is almost always benefit to narrowing your topic to be very specific for your project. This helps in naming the problem more clearly, using that name consistently to guide the literature review, considering project feasibility, and then projecting further clinical study plans. In essence, you are seeking movement from that fuzzy area of concern or "mess" to a clear problem statement and potential plan. Narrowing or funneling, seeing the change from a large global problem to a more concrete, detailed problem, helps focus the problem to a more doable clinical project topic. A funneling method, starting broadly and then narrowing the options, is done by continuing to ask whether a more narrow focus helps name this problem or issue more clearly, as well as leads to a more focused, useful project approach.

Related to the earlier example of a group dining setting in a long-term care facility your thoughts might proceed as follows. The group dining room situation is a "mess" and needs to function better. Determine, which patient groups are having the most challenges? Then, what does the literature say about working with these patient groups? Or perhaps you will determine another pathway to narrow the problem, such as staffing issues that seem to be problematic or staff needing further education. Then, which staff seem to have the most challenges helping patients or who could provide more help? What does the literature say about these issues, both in general and in long-term care dining settings?

Using another example, if you have determined the problem is a unit need for palliative care education, you still have a very broad statement with limited specifics about what that need is. Moving forward you would take this broad topic and determine specific educational needs for your focus. Sample approaches might be to narrow the topic to areas such as pain, symptom management, or family involvement in care. These concepts could be further explored and narrowed to the many areas, all within this broad problem, that could help improve patient care. When a range of options is identified, it becomes easier to focus on the specific needs for unit staff education and to further focus a project plan. As noted in the palliative care education example, most problems start broad and then need to be narrowed to have a much more specific, direct focus. Once you have narrowed the focus, it is easier to move forward in naming and packaging what you will do in your clinical project.

## Clarifying the Problem Name and Description

Why is clarifying the problem name important? Basically, you have to make sure that your project team and future readers know what you mean by the use of the selected term. You will have to confirm that others agree with this terminology and that your use of the term is consistent with how others (e.g., the literature) are using it. Even if your project becomes a broad exploratory approach to learn more about the problem, you will still need broad descriptors of the concept you are studying. Depending on the problem you choose to study, describing/defining is often considered similar to or a basic step of concept analysis, which is discussed in Chapter 7. Resources, such as the work of Walker and Avant (2019), provide further details.

If you are concerned, for example, about the problem of increasing incidence of delirium in healthcare settings, first you will need to define and describe what is meant by "delirium." How does the best evidence or literature define and use the term? If you wish to pursue a project that includes palliative care education, you will need to further define what the term "palliative care" means; for example, differentiating or identifying similarities and differences from the concept of hospice. Note also that you have indicated the concept of education as a part of the problem solution. For a scholarly project, you need to further describe what the concept of education means. Two basic questions to address are: What are you naming your concepts? How are you defining your concepts for study? This will include clarifying what the concepts are as well as what they are not, and then using that name and its definition consistently as you move forward.

## Describing Context and Setting Boundaries

What makes the problem context and the problem boundaries important considerations? Part of naming and defining the problem includes putting the chosen problem in a selected setting and identifying the problem boundaries for purposes of the project. Context is the broad setting, and the boundaries establish what is included in and excluded from that context.

Describing the context of a project includes helping others better understand the people, place, and process factors related to your project. Providing the right amount of detail (e.g., describing that the project is set in an emergency department in a small rural hospital versus a large urban medical center) helps others understand your project context. This is particularly useful to others in helping to determine whether a similar project might work in their settings.

Naming or setting the boundaries helps you and your reader understand what you are doing, as well as what are you not doing related to this problem. Stating, for example, that $x$ will be included in the project but $y$ will not helps identify the boundaries of the problem you plan to study and frames the problem to more clearly identify where it starts and stops. This also helps limit the extraneous issues and extraneous data, making the project clearer and more manageable. For example, which of the following provides more focus?

- The context/boundaries for this project are all elderly patients in this hospital with risk factors for delirium.
- The context/boundaries for this project are patients with a dementia diagnosis on a specific surgical unit who are at risk for delirium.

Note that the second statement provides more direction. The intent is to further narrow and determine what is most important and most feasible or practical to include in the project (Leedy & Ormrod, 2019). In simple terms, this means putting a frame or boundary around the topic/problem/issue you are addressing and then describing the surrounding factors. The Standards for Quality Improvement Reporting Excellence (2015) resources provide additional discussion about this topic.

## WHAT MAKES THIS A GOOD AND IMPORTANT PROBLEM TO STUDY?

What makes your problem an important one to study? Why is this problem significant to others? Does it matter or make a contribution to practice? Does it address a practical, clinical concern? Use the following additional questions (Leedy & Ormrod, 2019) to guide your thinking during development and write up of the problem statement:

1. Is the problem of current interest? Is it topical?
2. Is the problem likely to continue into the future?
3. Will more information about the problem have practical or theoretical applications?
4. How large is the population affected by the problem?
5. How would study of this problem lead to improving the problem or extend existing knowledge about the problem?
6. Would clinical project findings potentially lead to some useful change in best practice?
7. Is there current research or evidence that supports the need for further study of this problem?

## INTRODUCING THE PROBLEM IN THE PROPOSAL

This is the time to make a case for the importance of your particular problem and the need to do the project. The following sections including problem significance, fine-tuning the problem, and common challenges provide direction.

### Problem Significance

Discussion of the problem significance provides the rationale for why you are taking on the project. Much of the challenge is articulating the specific clinical problems and challenges so that others understand them. Here you introduce and make the case for the importance of the problem you want to address. This includes (a) describing the background of the problem; (b) addressing broad issues by providing a brief summary of current knowledge of the problem being addressed in broad populations or organizations; (c) addressing local issues by describing the nature and severity of the specific local problem or system dysfunction to be addressed; (d) and finally, summarizing a specific statement of the problem to be addressed in the project. This problem statement then leads to identifying the project purpose, setting the stage for determining best methods to guide the project.

### Fine-Tuning the Problem Statement

The problem statement serves to describe the important issues or conditions that exist in leading to the proposed project. An effective problem statement names the extent of the problem and supporting evidence, identifies factors contributing to the situation, and notes current gaps in addressing the problem (Coley et al., 2021).

Although the background of the problem is described in multiple paragraphs, a specific statement comprising several sentences that summarize the problem is beneficial to you in clearly naming the problem as well as communicating its significance to others. This statement clearly identifies your area of concern as a specific problem and provides a clear name of the issue you plan to focus on. It names what the problem is and clarifies what it is not. The problem statement is part of the first section of the proposal and introduces the reader to your problem. After reading your summary of the problem, ask yourself the following:

- Can I clearly answer the question: "What is the problem?"
- Is the scope appropriately limited with a balance of completeness and conciseness?
- Can I state why this problem is important and why it is worthy of a project?
- Does the problem summary place the specific problem in the context of the larger world?
- Does it describe the problem as important and interesting?
- Does the problem statement set the stage for a reasonable and feasible project to follow?

### Common Challenges With Problem Statements

After a fine-tuning of your problem statement, it should clearly and concisely identify the clinical problem your project will address, as well as its context. Review your problem statement and make sure it avoids the following common mistakes:

- The problem is not clearly stated or is vague and lost in discussion of broad, general issues.
- Components that contribute to the problem are not well identified or addressed.
- Limited or weak data are presented to support the problem importance (and not logically organized).
- The problem is not stated consistently.
- There is limited interest or need for study of the suggested problem.
- The problem is not framed in an adequate context (Leedy & Ormrod, 2019).
- The problem does not lead to a feasible project.

### Peer Review of Problem Statements

Again, recall the value of peer/mentor review. Discussing the problem statement (and other project components) with others can help you improve your work. As you review the following example problem statements, determine whether the problem statement is well focused and is specific enough to provide direction for a project. If you were completing a peer review for a colleague, do the following two problem-statement summaries provide beginning project direction? Which provides the most direction? What details would you recommend adding to either statement?

- Standardized electronic health record (EHR) documentation helps meet clinical, legal, and payment requirements. EHRs improve communication and efficiency in gaining patient information and documenting patient encounters. In reviewing the literature, few studies were found related to staff challenges and attitudes toward implementing a new EHR documentation system. A problem exists in helping staff best accept and prepare to use new EHR systems.

- College students are a unique population. College is an important transition time, and the health behaviors students choose in college often set the stage for lifetime health behaviors. A problem exists in helping students gain motivation and action toward improved health behaviors.

Note that both statements could be improved with more specific supporting data, such as literature and report references, that help make the case. Further context could be added to help identify the project needs locally as well. Further clarification of terms, such as what is meant by "health behaviors," would also be indicated.

## Using the Title to Help Convey the Project Intent

The project title is the most read component of the project. Clearly naming the problem and approaches within the project title can promote project clarity. To begin, this includes thinking about and naming what the problem is and what it is not. For example, if you are naming a problem related to staff development for older adult care, there is a lot of variation between the problem "need for improved care of the frail elderly" versus "promoting wellness for older adults." These concepts lead to two very different pathways for a project. Both can be of value, but early work on the project title can better guide the project. The correct name contributes to or sets the path for a good project. As you move forward with your purpose or aims statement, try writing a possible title to help focus your project direction.

Incorporating the problem into the *project title* is only one component of a well-chosen title. When your project purpose and methods take shape, they will influence the title as well. As your problem statement progresses and you move into the purpose statement phase, you will begin to think about the overarching title of your project and how to incorporate project approaches. Being able to state clearly in your title what you are going to do can help state your intent. Do not overstate what your proposed project can accomplish. Peer review could include asking others what they think your title conveys. Additionally review titles of previous DNP projects and note which are the clearest examples; you can find examples at www.doctorsofnursingpractice.org/doctoral-project-repository/

Once you have clearly identified the project problem, you are ready to use components of the project triangle model to develop your proposal.

## Project Triangle

It is not too early to start getting the points of the project triangle to align. After the problem is clearly named and described, use of the project triangle begins. The problem statement then leads to developing your project purpose, so it is important that it is well thought out and used consistently throughout the entire project. This is important as you develop your outcomes and methods and determine their feasibility. For example, in a project intended to learn about staff issues with a new EHR system, a very simple project triangle might include the following:

- *Purpose*: Understand staff concerns and satisfaction with the new EHR system.
- *Methods*: Staff completes survey including questions on concerns and satisfaction.
- *Outcome*: Evidence for any needed staff development is gained.

For reference, this triangle is shown in Chapter 1 (Figure 1.1), and Appendix A at the end of the book.

The experience of DNP students who have preceded you in the proposal-writing process is valuable. Their advice is presented in the following box.

### ADVICE FROM DNP STUDENTS

**Problem Selection**

Narrow your topic as much as is reasonably possible:

- "The most difficult/challenging aspect was to narrow my topic."
- "Deciding on what aspect to focus on for my project was a challenge. There were so many different ways I could have gone."

Find a project idea you enjoy:

- "I really enjoy my topic, and so the time just flies by as I am trying to figure things out."

### PRACTICE SCHOLARSHIP APPLICATIONS

Consider your competency documentation plans. How will your project address select *Essentials*? Consider additions to your project notebook as you complete the following.

- *Concepts to competence*: What tools have you gained for documenting your problem statement? What is your self-assessment of your ability to move from a fuzzy problem to a clear problem statement?
- *Essentials*: Review advanced level competencies and subcompetencies for the *Essentials* domains Knowledge for Nursing Practice, Scholarship for Nursing Practice, and Quality and Safety, and reflect on how they relate to your planned DNP project.
- *Project notebook*: Start with a one-page written reflection that incorporates the process that is helping you identify and fine-tune your problem. Indicate the setting and mentor you plan to use (see the Learning Activities later in this chapter).

## SUMMARY AND KEY POINTS

Clinical problems with relevance for advanced clinical projects abound. The problem statement sets the stage or describes the status of a current situation that needs to be addressed. It serves as the background for project purpose statements. It helps if the problem statement emerges from strong personal interests and meets unit needs as well as promoting professional scholarship. This chapter offered direction in identifying important problems and focusing them for further study. Points to recall from this chapter include the following:

- Problem statements are based on areas of clinical concern and unit need.
- Put the problem in context, address where your project is happening and how you will access the site.
- Focus problem statements by narrowing the topic.
- Name the problem clearly and consistently.
- Set boundaries to establish the problem context.
- Fine-tune the problem statement to avoid common problems.
- Introduce your problem statement by establishing it significance.
- Convey information about the problem via a clear project title.

## WEBSITES FOR FURTHER REVIEW

Relating your problem to data from national reports can support the need for addressing the problem and help place it in context. For example, you may find it useful to relate your problem to changing demographics. Although the following reports are specific to issues of older adults and health disparities, similar reports can be found to describe other populations and issues. What surprises you as you review these reports? What ideas do you gain for helping document your clinical problems?

- *2019 Profile of Older Americans*:
  https://acl.gov/sites/default/files/Aging%20and%20Disability%20in%20America/2019ProfileOlderAmericans508.pdf
- *Retooling for an Aging America: Building the Health Care Workforce*:
  www.nationalacademies.org/hmd/reports/2008/retooling-for-an-aging-america-building-the-health-care-workforce.aspx
- *A Framework for Educating Health Professionals to Address the Social Determinants of Health*:
  www.nap.edu/catalog/21923/a-framework-for-educating-health-professionals-to-address-the-socialdeterminants-of-health

## NEXT CHAPTER UP

The goal of clinical projects is to improve practice. You now have a clearly crafted problem statement and, with this problem statement in hand, you are ready to delve more deeply into a project plan. The next chapter provides background on quality improvement and how it can help inform your next project decisions.

### ONLINE/CLASSROOM DISCUSSION

**Peer Review of Problem Statements**

Place yourself in the role of providing peer review for a colleague's clinical project problem statement. What suggestions would you make to your colleague for improving the following initial problem statements? What is missing from each? What ways might you rewrite these?

- Providing congestive heart failure (CHF) education is needed.
- Increasing the number of diabetic foot exams is important.
- Evaluating the effectiveness of inpatient stroke education is necessary.

## LEARNING ACTIVITIES

### For Your Project Notebook: Your Story Related to Your Topic of Interest

One way to begin developing a problem of interest is to write about it from a personal perspective. How is your story related to your topic of interest? Why is it important to you? What do you hope to accomplish? As you identify a problem of concern, write a few paragraphs about what it means to you and why it is important to you. This reflection can help focus the problem and provide an opportunity for you and faculty to communicate. For a specific problem that you have in mind, ask the following questions:

- What makes this problem important?
- Why does it matter? Are there important patient concerns? Staff concerns?
- As you consider the problem in context, are there staff approaches or processes that seem to work well? Processes that could work better?
- What potential contributions could be made from further studying or developing this project?

### Further Reflective-Writing Prompts

- I am choosing this topic because …
- It is important I do this project because …
- Challenges in taking on this topic include …
- Early findings from the literature review suggest …

## To-Do List

- Find three key articles that most help you make your case and move your project forward for the problem you would like to pursue.
- Identify and confirm a specific topic of concern that can be addressed by the clinical project.
- Write an introduction that presents the importance of your clinical problem and what is known about it. End the initial section of your proposal with a clear, one or two sentence problem statement that clarifies the problem and why it is important.

## Readiness to Proceed

- Have you started a literature review related to your problem?
- Have you tried to think about the problem from multiple angles and perspectives?
- Have you considered the pros and cons for addressing this problem?
- Have you thought about the feasibility of addressing this problem?
- Have you gained expert advice on strategies and challenges for your planned approach to the problem?

## REFERENCES

Coley, S., Scheinberg, C., & Strekalova, Y. (2021). *Proposal writing: Effective grantsmanship for funding* (6th ed.). Sage.

Krathwohl, D., & Smith, N. (2005). *How to prepare a dissertation proposal: Suggestions for students in education and the social and behavioral sciences.* Syracuse University Press.

Leedy, P., & Ormrod, J. (2019). *Practical research: Planning and design* (12th ed.). Pearson.

Standards for Quality Improvement Reporting Excellence. (2015). *Revised standards for quality improvement reporting excellence, SQUIRE 2.0.* http://www.squire-statement.org/index.cfm?fuseaction=Page.ViewPage&PageID=471

Walker, L., & Avant, K. (2019). *Strategies for theory construction in nursing* (6th ed.). Prentice Hall.

# 4. Clinical Projects and Quality Improvement: Thinking "Big Picture"

## INITIAL THOUGHT

"Isn't quality improvement what a good project is all about?"

## CHAPTER CONTENT

- Reflective Questions
- Quality Improvement Alert
- How Can Clinical Projects Help Improve Practice?
- Is Your Project a Match for Quality Improvement?
- Quality Improvement: Systems and Population Perspectives
  - Thinking Systems
  - Thinking Populations
- Systems and Population Perspective Examples
- Quality Improvement: Problem-Solving and Needs Assessments
  - Needs Assessments
  - Documenting Need From the Literature
  - Addressing the Root Cause
  - Sharing Focused Descriptive Reports
  - Technology and Large Data Sets as Points of Needs Assessments
  - Using SWOT Tools
  - Checklists as Quality Improvement Resources
- Practice Scholarship Applications
- Summary and Key Points
- Websites for Further Review
- Next Chapter Up
- Online/Classroom Discussion
- Learning Activities
  - Gaining Skills: Developing Big-Picture Ideas Related to Your Topic of Interest
  - Planning Activity: Building on Your Own Quality Improvement Experiences
  - Planning Activity: Learning From Others
  - To-Do List/Readiness to Proceed

## REFLECTIVE QUESTIONS

In Chapter 3, you learned about ideas for thinking and naming a clinical problem. Now the focus is on the big picture of projects, many influenced by the quality-improvement (QI) perspective. This chapter provides background on how QI can help inform your project decisions as well as strategies to help document the need for your project on a local practice level. The following reflective questions organize learning for this chapter. Which of the following are you most confident?

- What is your perspective on how clinical projects help improve practice?
- How can understanding QI lead to potential project frames?
- How does describing systems models and population perspectives relate to QI?
- What are the practical approaches to beginning QI data collection and analysis for needs assessments?

Use the Practice Scholarship Applications (at the end of this chapter) to help document your learning from concept to competency, including the relevant American Association of Colleges of Nursing (AACN) *Essentials* (2021).

## QUALITY IMPROVEMENT ALERT

Having a good understanding of QI is relevant to good problem-solving, from needs assessment to a completed durable project. This chapter introduces the QI process with a focus on needs assessments.

## HOW CAN CLINICAL PROJECTS HELP IMPROVE PRACTICE?

QI and clinical application scholarship go hand in hand. QI is also a key *Essentials* component. The goal of clinical projects is to improve practice. This chapter focuses on QI and needs assessments. Additional chapters in this book focus on methods used in the project implementation and evaluation phases of QI projects.

Now that you have identified an important clinical problem, this chapter summarizes big-picture approaches to help you gain focus for your clinical project. Although numerous approaches to clinical projects exist, QI is typically an underlying theme. These QI projects provide the opportunity to combine scholarly evidence with a local clinical problem or issue. This chapter helps you think about potential project opportunities within the QI frame as you begin to move from a problem area to a project idea.

## IS YOUR PROJECT A MATCH FOR QUALITY IMPROVEMENT?

QI models provide guidance that can improve patient care. QI has long been an important topic as it documents a type of accountability in healthcare. It takes on increasing importance now with the current focus on safety and quality care needs, as documented in national error reports. Once you have identified a problem, then the focus becomes trying to fix that problem. You can ask whether a QI focus would work for you as you move into the big picture of mapping your project. For example, you might be aware of best-evidence literature indicating that preoperative patient education programs for joint replacements help improve patient outcomes. If you feel this could be an important issue in your setting, would this be the type of QI project you would want to pursue?

From a practical perspective, QI means gaining and maintaining quality processes and products in healthcare, with a focus on safe, quality care for patients. QI is considered a problem-solving process that uses a model to guide its process. As an ongoing process, it incorporates quality process and outcome indicators (American Public Health Association, 2013). QI brings useful models for considering the big picture and documenting specific agency or community needs as an initial component of project planning. Points to consider are as follows:

- QI incorporates a systems perspective. It is important to understand systems because most healthcare agencies can be considered from a systems perspective. As national error reports indicate, many safety concerns occur because these systems are not working as they should.
- QI involves a reflective component. You will reflect and then ask questions about problems or challenges that you are seeing. As a reflective reader of other QI projects related to your problem of interest, you learn about strategies that others have tried. You reflect and ask whether a particular evidence-based protocol might work in your setting or with your population of interest.
- QI involves teams. A good QI project should be an example of good teamwork. A project might engage unit members to implement a new initiative; for example, engaging the team in implementing and evaluating a new care model or communication protocol. QI projects can help engage staff to take accountability for the big picture of care.
- QI involves feedback and ongoing monitoring. Once a project is implemented, you will want to know whether it works. Consistent with a problem-solving model, QI involves evaluation of the project and then feedback to the team. Ongoing project monitoring helps ensure needed improvements are sustained.

A variety of continuous QI models exist, as further noted in Chapter 7. Detailed approaches to organizing and documenting QI, such as the Standards for Quality Improvement Reporting Excellence (2015) resource, are also available.

## QUALITY IMPROVEMENT: SYSTEMS AND POPULATION PERSPECTIVES

As part of QI, understanding systems and populations helps to determine project needs and to describe clearly the project of interest. Many projects start at the micro-system, or smaller unit, level. A pilot project can be used to identify the project challenges and successes within a small population or one hospital unit. When beginning a project, it is especially important to identify for oneself and others what system is to be used and who will be the population of interest.

Naming systems and populations can also help outline what you are interested in and why. For example, if you are hoping to improve diabetes care for patient populations in your practice setting, a QI approach could be one consideration. You would review the literature for the best evidence. Then you might consider using that evidence to develop a checklist approach for chart audits regarding team adherence to best diabetes care practices. If that review indicates a gap or lack of consistency in implementing best practices in your setting, and patient population outcomes are not reaching standards, then feedback to the team and engaging an improvement plan are indicated. This can then lead to the next steps of a QI project to help improve that care.

### Thinking Systems

Systems models describe the organizations that play a central role in healthcare. Systems perspectives incorporate a network of interdependent components, allowing an opportunity to view patterns and relationships versus individual issues (Nelson et al., 2008). Big-picture thinking provides the opportunity to identify a system's success and challenges and to consider how these impact safe, quality care (Johnson et al., 2008). Points to recall about systems and why they are important include the following:

- National safety reports expound on the need to improve healthcare systems and create a culture of safety. Placing a specified problem in the context of a designated system helps one better understand the problem and identify where specific system changes (such as new unit policies and procedures) are needed.
- Systems models, credited to Donabedian (1988), provide a reasonable framework for thinking about diverse

issues within the broad concepts of structure, process, and outcomes. These concepts help characterize the organization or specific agency unit and help convey the interdependent nature of people, place, and process. *Structure* involves how things are organized. For example, a specific unit, such as a rehab unit, can be described in terms of its structure (staff, resources, and setting). *Process* is the way things are done (protocols, steps for accomplishing the work of a unit). *Outcomes* are the products you are seeking to attain (the desired accomplishments).

- To understand and improve outcomes, as well as to share what a project has accomplished, it is important to describe the structure and process that go with these outcomes.

## Thinking Populations

Naming and describing your population characteristics are important components of your QI project. Diverse populations are noted to include clinical populations, community populations, or other aggregates (American Association of Colleges of Nursing, 2006). Populations incorporate diverse considerations, including health dimensions, culture, socioeconomics, and environment. Documenting the population and its health is important in acute care, primary care, long-term care, and public health (Institute of Medicine, 2012). Cultivating a better understanding of a particular population can be important to clinical projects in multiple ways:

- In a primary care setting, describing subpopulations can help identify potential issues within the larger primary care population. Knowing subpopulation issues, for example, the patient aggregate engaged with family caregiving and its related challenges, can lead to better opportunities to address these concerns. Strategies to facilitate the care of this subpopulation can then emerge. For example, caregiver screening tools for individuals caring for loved ones with dementia might be implemented to identify caregiver risk for healthcare issues. Knowing the demographics of populations and subpopulations can then help identify not only needs for practice policies and procedures, but further needs in education and research.

- Comparisons of populations can also be useful in health-promotion efforts. For example, knowing the characteristics of your community in terms of the extent of the risk for hypertension or stroke, and then learning that your community has higher percentages of these cardiac diagnoses compared with state and national data, leads you to ask "Why is this happening?" You might also wonder what approaches other communities have taken to improve similar problems and review resources to gain ideas for your community.

- A population focus can remind you to compare data and learn from others dealing with similar situations. As noted, often large respected national resources such as the Centers for Disease Control and Prevention and Healthy People 2030 are useful in making comparisons between local populations and state or national populations. This can help support documentation and context for a local need.

## SYSTEMS AND POPULATION PERSPECTIVE EXAMPLES

Systems and population concepts can lead to ideas for developing a project. Thinking of the population and systems helps consider the project's components, including potential needs and challenges. Relevant DNP project examples include the following:

- A DNP student, working at a primary care clinic, found their practice was seeing many patients with chronic kidney disease (CKD) and its related risks (Appendix C). The student was not sure that the clinic was using best evidence in guiding patient care for this subpopulation. The student project used a best-evidence checklist, developed from their literature review, to complete chart audits. After analyzing the data, the student then compared the audit findings to the current best-evidence recommendations to identify practice strengths and gaps. These were shared with staff for QI.

- A DNP student, in their work at a mental health center clinic (Appendix D), found that a large percentage of the patient population was dealing with diabetes. The student proposed a QI project that reviewed clinic records to better address care needs for this population. The student's findings helped identify gaps in care, propose improvements in documentation, and implement use of a checklist as a tool for improving delivery of care to meet American Diabetes Association standards.

- In a hospital setting, another DNP student (Appendix E) felt that unit-based councils were a good strategy to engage staff in quality care. After these councils were put in place at a select organization, the student wanted to confirm that nursing staff and managers agreed that these councils were useful as part of their healthcare system. The student's QI project focused on staff perspectives of the unit-based councils' effectiveness as well as their challenges. The results were shared with agency staff for QI.

In each of these examples, reflections and questions specific to a local practice concern led to ideas that could help improve quality care more broadly. The projects, using QI principles included systems thinking and a population focus to address practice concerns. Further QI principles for the projects included engaging staff to first better understand the problem and then generate plans to help improve specific outcomes.

## QUALITY IMPROVEMENT: PROBLEM-SOLVING AND NEEDS ASSESSMENTS

QI approaches address a pressing clinical issue in terms of solving a problem or improving care. Improvement projects are planned to help promote safe clinical care delivery and enhanced patient outcomes. Typically, the project scope is narrow and the context is a specified unit or setting. The project integrates appropriate use of literature-based best evidence with real-world practice.

Problem-solving approaches are a part of QI and include addressing the need for a select project. Needs assessments, an important component of problem-solving, provide data that can help describe and convey to others the baseline system and population issues. This provides a way to name and more clearly understand problems or gaps in care, as well as providing baseline data used to seek improvement. Approaches to needs assessments vary, with both detailed approaches that might become a clinical project itself, or more basic approaches that use quickly available data to outline a basic need for a QI project.

### Needs Assessments

Needs assessments help to name and document current situations in preparation for making improvements. They can help those interested in understanding the who, what, and when of a problem, providing the context for a project. Note that your broad literature review addresses the extent of the problem from a professional body of knowledge, whereas the local needs assessment provides the local context of the problem you are addressing.

Needs assessments can be extensive, detailed projects in themselves, or practical assessments made primarily with available data, to show the need for QI. Needs assessments provide the opportunity to gain new data to help clarify a problem or help generate evidence about gaps in evidence-based practices that currently exist. These are often the first step in a larger project, such as a new program in a community or hospital setting. Sometimes a systems model helps frame a needs assessment, that is, asking questions to determine structures and processes that currently exist and then considering how a new proposed program could build on or add to this for improved outcomes. Broad questions to address in a needs assessment include the following:

- Who/what are the people, the places, and process factors important in your future project?
- What methods can be used to identify the key needs of this entity or the cause of the clinical issue/problem (i.e., fishbone diagram)?
- How does the proposed project fit with the organization or community's goals?

In considering this broad approach with a clinical problem example in a long-term care setting, the issue might include older adult challenges, such as not eating well in a group dining setting. A further developed needs assessment gained from either formal or informal interviews and observations with staff and residents could help document the problem in greater detail. Paired with a review of the literature to gain ideas from other clinical scholars' work, documenting need for change could help in solving components of the problem.

As you begin to think about the big picture of your project, confirm that you can document the need for the project. To start this process, think about data that you can easily access that will help you describe a local system or a population's specific needs. Many QI tools exist to help extend the basic who, what, how, and when, which often guide a quick assessment. Sample approaches involved in needs assessment include documenting the need as described in the literature, root cause analyses, focused descriptive reports, large data sets, and SWOT (strengths/weaknesses/opportunities/threats) analyses.

### Documenting Need From the Literature

When you first identify a clinical problem, you then move to the literature hoping to find evidence-based strategies that others have used to successfully resolve a problem similar to yours. Sometimes you find syntheses of evidence or national reports that have addressed your issue; they may have reviewed successful strategies or made recommendations for further testing. These can provide a national scholarly perspective that you can then compare with your local problem for similarities and differences.

Especially in a new problem area, one with limited study, your literature review and synthesis can be a major component of helping document needs for further work in a clinical area. One leadership student wished to develop a nursing alumnae association but found there was limited literature on this topic. She moved to a project that included a systematic review of university websites and interviews with other leaders who had already developed this resource (Birk, 2015). Another student was interested in developing a rural health clinic and found the literature provided limited evidence on how best to do this. She then moved forward to a descriptive evidence-generating project, completing interviews and learning from rural nurse practitioners experienced with these clinics (Appendix F).

### Addressing the Root Cause

Analyzing the cause of clinical issues or events using a root cause analysis can contribute to broad needs assessments, leading to better understanding of a problem or issue to be addressed. Diagramming potential causative factors of a problem can be an early step in understanding and then resolving the problem. Flowchart-type diagrams help map a procedure or process to help identify where a process might break down. Fishbone diagrams provide graphic outlines of potential concepts or factors that contribute to a problem. These diagramming techniques can help you identify where to start in naming a problem or may help you rename or refocus a particular problem.

A good example showing the fishbone diagram in action, is provided in the National Action Plan for Adverse Drug Event Prevention (ADE Action Plan). Using the fishbone diagram, authors identified where potential challenges related to the problem might be found. This included diagramming the concepts of provider, patient, and proximate factors, as well as the impact of the healthcare system, including technical and latent factors, with potential impact on adverse drug reactions (https://health.gov/hcq/pdfs/ade-action-plan-508c.pdf).

This diagramming then provides the opportunity for further assessment and planning at the local level. Incorporating the "Five Ws" (i.e., asking "why" five times) in the root cause analysis can also help to begin or delve more deeply into a problem, ensuring that you address the problem at the level where it exists. Other examples using a fishbone diagram are provided by the Institute for Healthcare Improvement, documenting challenges with long wait times for lab results (www.ihi.org/sites/default/files/SafetyToolkit_Causeand EffectDiagram.pdf).

### Sharing Focused Descriptive Reports

A focused descriptive report involves describing and reporting a specified clinical context in a meaningful way. Often applications for clinical agency designations, such as a center for excellence, rehabilitation specialty unit, or a cancer center, require documents similar or equivalent to needs assessments. Agencies may have completed recent reports with needs assessments that could help document your needs assessment or provide further context for the problem identified.

In addition, community and population needs assessments are often indicated for a particular project. One student, for example, interested in supporting older adults in their homes, completed a needs survey related to community services for older adults to better identify resources and gaps. After completing the assessment, the student identified the need for an older adult transportation program, and then generated a plan to engage faith communities in a service project related to this need. Another individual, in preparation for developing an onsite clinic, completed a needs assessment of an assisted living facility, documenting and describing the people, the setting, and their processes for gaining clinical care. These data helped identify baseline information as well as document gaps and needs for developing the clinic project.

### Technology and Large Data Sets as Points of Needs Assessments

Information technologies such as Typhon are not new for data reporting, but they can be a valuable tool to help tell the story of your practice populations. As you learn primary care of individual patients, consider opportunities to gain a populations perspective of your practice. This needs assessment includes the addition of reflective questions to electronic graphic reports of clinical logs. Enhancing your traditional clinical log by running and graphing your data reports can help you describe your practice, identify practice needs, make practice change recommendations, and identify topics for future clinical project needs. In one example, a student used the graphing function on their Typhon report to group and identify their patients' diagnoses and payment methods. This led to helping document the practice need for more attention to patients with diabetes who were also using Medicaid services.

### Using SWOT Tools

A SWOT analysis can be a useful component of project planning. This tool provides the opportunity to better understand an issue within the context of your population and setting before developing a project. The four SWOT concepts provide guidance for mapping a clinical problem within a unit. This approach helps to focus on a clinical unit's positives and take advantage of its strengths, and map challenges or areas needing to be improved. For example, in creating a needs assessment to prepare for a specialty unit certification, a DNP student completed a SWOT analysis, which led to projecting potential QI projects to consider (Exhibit 4.1).

### Checklists as Quality Improvement Resources

Another way of thinking about a needs assessment is an appropriate checklist to help document quality approaches to care. Checklists take many forms and can be used in diverse ways. In general, they are intended to help minimize human factor errors and help providers have confidence in the processes they are completing. Good clinical checklists or algorithms are determined from the best evidence on a topic/procedure and require appropriate validation of design, content, and process for use (Agency for Healthcare Research and Quality [AHRQ], 2010). Although checklists are not always used as a needs assessment, they have that potential. In the proposal example in Appendix C, the student used a checklist from the literature to audit practice charts and determine practice compliance or gaps in using best practices specific to chronic kidney disease. Results led to further QI opportunities for the practice.

> **EXHIBIT 4.1 SWOT EXAMPLE: NEEDS ASSESSMENT AS PART OF A PROJECT PLAN FOR SPECIALTY-UNIT CERTIFICATION**
>
> **Brigid Weyhofen**
>
> *Purpose*
>
> Purpose is to prepare for a clinical unit excellence application (seeking unit specialty certification). Three key areas were addressed: (a) compliance with national standards, (b) evidence-based clinical practice guidelines, and (c) performance measures (comprehensive care for joint-replacement patients, bundled payments for joint replacements, and provider responsible for patient 90 days postoperatively). The certification for joint excellence application focuses on documenting quality care, continuous improvement outcomes, and good stewardship of resources.
>
> *Clinical Unit Current Status*
>
> *Strengths*: Established joint replacement program, engaged nursing leadership and attending physician with interest in improving outcomes. Hospital has a unit that has been designated for joint replacement patients. Academic medical setting.
>
> *Weaknesses*: Lack of training/education for nursing staff, limited means for collection of data, lack of planning of surgery schedule with bed placement, complex surgery schedule with delayed cases, limited physical therapy resources, payor source limits home resources, need for improved communication, and inconsistent preoperative education.
>
> *Opportunities*: Increase market share, decrease the percentage of joint replacement readmissions, increase nurse retention, decrease lengths of stay, and increase preoperative education for patients.
>
> *Threats*: Reimbursement changes, ongoing financial support need, competing priorities in an organization.
>
> *Initial and Ongoing Strategies for This "Preparation" Journey*
>
> *Engaging key stakeholders*: Relationship building, planning/goal setting, improved communication, partnering, stakeholder education, joint unit excellence requirements.
>
> *Education for staff*: Identification of key staff members, workday to develop care pathway, development of basic "joint" class for all.
>
> *Sample Process Improvement Projects Evolving From This SWOT*
>
> From this preliminary work and needs/SWOT analysis, sample process improvement projects emerged. Examples include
>
> - improved time from postanesthesia care unit to floor,
> - improved preoperative education for patients, and
> - improved patient's perception of readiness for discharge.

---

> **PRACTICE SCHOLARSHIP APPLICATIONS**
>
> Consider your competency documentation plans. How will your project address select *Essentials*? Consider additions to your project notebook as you complete the following.
>
> - *Concepts to competence*: What tools have you gained for using a quality improvement approach to your project? Review the questions from the beginning of this chapter and self-assess on your progress.
> - *Essentials*: Review advanced evaluation competencies and subcompetencies for the Quality and Safety; Systems-Based Practice; and Interprofessional Partnerships *Essentials* domains, and reflect on how they relate to your clinical project.
> - *Project notebook*: Include a one-page written reflection on your own QI efforts related to your project. Address the process that is helping you gain populations and systems-based QI perspectives.

## SUMMARY AND KEY POINTS

Recall that this chapter addressed QI broadly and needs assessments specifically. Future chapters include implementation evaluation phases to develop the QI project. QI approaches are a staple in healthcare; they provide systems and population perspectives. They also provide a structure and process for outlining problem approaches and monitoring quality, as well as reminding us of the importance of documenting project needs. They provide tools for naming the big picture of clinical challenges and then framing potential projects. Chapter 16 provides further discussion related to implementing an evidence-based QI project. Points to recall from this chapter include the following:

- Consider the QI frame for a clinical project that can be designed to help improve clinical practice.
- In general, QI is considered a type of problem-solving model, with a focus on systems, populations, teams, feedback, and monitoring.
- Problem-solving approaches, such as QI, incorporate needs assessment tools such as root cause analyses, SWOT analyses, checklists, literature reviews, and descriptive reports.
- Considering populations and subpopulations reminds us to name and describe the populations or subpopulations the project is designed to serve.

- Systems and population perspectives are important in QI, reminding us to add the big picture and context of a project.
- Practical considerations as you begin QI projects include incorporating problem-solving models.

## WEBSITES FOR FURTHER REVIEW

These are some examples of resources used to gain more information about QI, offering further ideas for the next steps:

- *Institute for Healthcare Improvement Quality Improvement Essentials Toolkit*:

    www.ihi.org/resources/tools/quality-improvement-essentials-toolkit

- *Quality Improvement*:

    www.ruralcenter.org/sites/default/files/HRSAQIToolkit.pdf

- *Standards for Quality Improvement Reporting Excellence* (in addition to detailed guidelines for outlining and reporting a QI project, project examples can be found within this site):

    www.squire-statement.org

## NEXT CHAPTER UP

You have reviewed a variety of concepts relevant to QI projects, including thinking about your project need at the local level. Now head to the literature to determine how others have approached the problem. The focus in the following two chapters includes reviewing and synthesizing the professional literature so that you can situate your project within that domain.

### ONLINE/CLASSROOM DISCUSSION

**Project Titles**

From a selection of potential project titles, which QI project titles are clearest to you? What QI approach is suggested? What are the populations and/or settings conveyed? What would you suggest to improve the following titles?

- *Implementing Evidence-Based Practice Guidelines for Diabetic Foot Screening*
- *Mental Health Workflow Integration in an Orthopedic Clinic for Adults*
- *Developing a Systematic Patient Safety Risk Assessment Tool to Prioritize Patient Safety Program Activities*
- *Developing Evidence-Based Education Material to Assist Older Adults With Swallowing Disorders*
- *Identifying Factors Contributing to Postdischarge Appointment Attendance*

## LEARNING ACTIVITIES

### Gaining Skills: Developing Big-Picture Ideas Related to Your Topic of Interest

Consider a potential clinic, agency, or population for your clinical project. Working with your clinical partners, how will you address the following questions?

- How will you describe this clinic as "an entity" or "a system?"
- What can you learn from asking the typical who, what, when, and where questions? What can you learn from a more detailed assessment?
- What are the obvious strengths and challenges you note with this agency or population?
- What ideas do you have for how this system might be improved? What priorities for change would you suggest (Johnson et al., 2008)?

### Planning Activity: Building on Your Own Quality Improvement Experiences

- What roles and responsibilities have you identified related to QI and patient care? What gaps exist in your knowledge of QI? What learning needs do you still have related to QI?
- What are some examples of how you have participated in or evaluated others' QI projects? What did you learn from those experiences? What strategies might serve you in a future QI project?
- What ideas do you have for your own QI project?

### Planning Activity: Learning From Others

- *Agency for Healthcare Research and Quality (AHRQ) Falls Prevention Toolkit*: The AHRQ website provides a falls toolkit (www.ahrq.gov/sites/default/files/publications/files/fallpxtoolkit.pdf) that lays out sample questions to ask as part of QI project planning. Documents such as this may direct you to components needed for your project plan. After reviewing the table of contents, select sections on the AHRQ Falls Prevention Toolkit for further review. What ideas from this large-scale project do you think might be useful to QI in your practice area?
- *AHRQ Health Literacy Universal Precautions Toolkit*: The AHRQ website also provides a Health Literacy Universal Precautions Toolkit (www.ahrq.gov/professionals/quality-patient-safety/quality-resources/tools/literacy-toolkit/index.html) with an array of resources for QI planning related to the concept of health

literacy. After reviewing the contents, select sections on this resource for further review. What ideas from this large-scale project might be useful to QI in your area of interest?

## To-Do List/Readiness to Proceed

During the early preparation for your project proposal, what do you think about the following?

- Is the problem/project a good match for a QI project?
- Have you considered the systems that will be used and the population that will be addressed in your project?
- Do you have plans for a good needs assessment and/or procuring baseline data specific to your problem of concern and potential project ideas?

## REFERENCES

Agency for Healthcare Research and Quality. (2010). *What makes a good checklist?* https://psnet.ahrq.gov/perspectives/perspective/92/what-makes-a-good-checklist

American Association of Colleges of Nursing. (2006). *The essentials of doctoral education for advanced nursing practice.* https://www.aacnnursing.org/DNP/DNP-Essentials

American Public Health Association. (2013). *Quality improvement in action.* https://www.apha.org/~/media/files/pdf/factsheets/qualityimprovement_fact_sheet.ashx

Birk, S. (2015). *The planning of a nurse alumni association: Gaining best evidence.* University of Kansas DNP Project.

Donabedian, A. (1988). The quality of care: How can it be assessed? *Journal of the American Medical Association, 260*(12), 1743–1748. https://doi.org/10.1001/jama.260.12.1743

Institute for Quality Improvement. (2017). *Quality improvement essentials toolkit.* Institute for Healthcare Improvement. https://www.ihi.org/resources/tools/quality-improvement-essentials-toolkit

Institute of Medicine. (2012). *Living well with chronic illness: A call for public health action.* National Academies Press.

Johnson, J., Miller, S., & Horowitz, S. (2008). *Systems-based practice: Improving the safety and quality of patient care by recognizing and improving the systems in which we work.* Agency for Healthcare Research and Quality.

Nelson, E., Godfrey, M. M., Batalden, P. B., Berry, S. A., Bothe, A. E., Jr., McKinley, K. E., Melin, C. N., Muething, S. E., Moore, L. G., Wasson, J. H., & Nolan, T. W. (2008). Clinical microsystems, part 1. The building blocks of health systems. *Joint Commission on Accreditation of Healthcare Organizations, 34*(7), 367–378. https://doi.org/10.1016/s1553-7250(08)34047-1

Standards for Quality Improvement Reporting Excellence. (2015). *Revised standards for quality improvement reporting excellence, SQUIRE 2.0.* http://www.squire-statement.org/index.cfm?fuseaction=Page.ViewPage&PageID=471

# 5. Into the Literature: Gaining Best Evidence and Relevant Literature

## INITIAL THOUGHT

"What does it take to be 'the best?'"

## CHAPTER CONTENT

- Reflective Questions
- Quality Improvement Alert
- What Makes a Good Literature Review?
- Literature Review as the Basis for Further Proposal Work
- Beginning the Literature Review
- Clarify the Type of Review
- Formal Systematic Reviews of the Literature: The Process Overview
- The Literature Search: Obtaining Evidence
  - Databases
  - Key Words
  - Inclusion/Exclusion Criteria
  - Practical/Methodological Screens
  - Primary/Secondary Sources
- Advice From DNP Students
- Challenges/Facilitators to Gaining the Evidence
  - What if You Cannot Find Research/Literature Evidence?
  - What if Accessing or Obtaining the Evidence Is Problematic?
  - What if You Have Trouble Keeping Track of the Search Process?
- Reading and Critiquing the Evidence
  - To Help in Reading
  - To Help in Evaluating the Quality of the Evidence
- The Evidence Summary: Organizing the Literature Review Findings
  - Archiving and Cataloguing
  - Reference Matrix
    - *Reference Matrix Format*
    - *Final Touches to the Reference Matrix*
  - Documenting Sources
- Literature Review Tips for Getting Started
- Practice Scholarship Applications
- Summary and Key Points
- Websites for Further Review
- Next Chapter Up
- Online/Classroom Discussion
- Learning Activities
  - To-Do List

## REFLECTIVE QUESTIONS

In Chapter 3, you learned about writing a good clinical problem. Now your focus is on finding the best evidence about that problem so that you can establish what is already known about it and what still needs to be determined. The following reflective questions organize learning for this chapter. With which of the following are you most confident?

- What makes a good systematic literature review?
- What type of literature review best suits your project proposal?
- What does "information literacy" mean to you and why is this relevant to your project proposal?
- What are the best strategies for completing a systematic literature review?
- What evidence makes the best evidence?
- What does it mean to complete a reference matrix?

Use the Practice Scholarship Applications (at the end of this chapter) to help document your learning from concept to competency, including the relevant American Association of Colleges of Nursing (AACN) *Essentials* (2021).

## QUALITY IMPROVEMENT ALERT

A formal literature review provides the most comprehensive context in which to conduct a research project, but scoping reviews often provide sufficient context for a quality improvement (QI) project.

## WHAT MAKES A GOOD LITERATURE REVIEW?

A good literature review is one that is systematically conducted, documented, synthesized, and situated in the context of the professional literature. Your literature review can help you narrow your practice concern to best name the problem you are studying. The literature also provides ideas about how much your problem area has been studied and, depending on the extent of previous work, may help identify evidence-based solutions. Coping with the vast quantities of literature available involves more than an informal literature review. The review for your project should be systematic, covering important aspects of the topic, and be representative of the work that has been done. A systematic literature review can be combined with an annotated bibliography or reference matrix to help organize information. For example, if you are seeking the best evidence on caring for new patients with stroke on a rehabilitation unit in a hospital or other clinical setting, what is the best evidence available about that care in the literature? Your systematic review and reference matrix provide the basis for an evidence-based synthesis of this literature.

## LITERATURE REVIEW AS THE BASIS FOR FURTHER PROPOSAL WORK

Gaining awareness of existing knowledge regarding best practice is critical to a good clinical project proposal, and this requires systematic approaches to the literature review. The systematic literature review, as previously noted, should be done simultaneously with the development of your problem and purpose statements. Completing a systematic review of the literature during these two steps helps to narrow the problem, refine the purpose statement, gain project direction, and establish the need for the project.

As you write your problem statement, the review of literature familiarizes you with the best evidence that currently exists specific to your chosen problem. The literature review also helps describe the context for the specified problem and patient population. It should also be ongoing so that the references you describe in your project truly reflect the rapidly changing evidence for your specified subject, with preference for references published within the last 3 to 5 years (unless the source is recognized as a classic/historical publication). This implies that the literature should be consistently updated throughout the duration of the entire clinical project.

A systematic review of the literature also helps establish you as an expert in the area and enables you to demonstrate your command of the literature, best evidence, and gaps in knowledge related to your topic and its context. This means you know the key authors writing in your topic area, you know the existing knowledge base on the topic, and you are able to identify the strengths and weaknesses of the evidence related to your clinical problem.

Finally, gaining and synthesizing the evidence are part of the scholarship of advanced clinical practice. Your contribution to clinical scholarship is best made if situated within past and present knowledge in the area. Identifying gaps in the topic can help make the case for your additional project work. Exhibit 5.1 provides a summary of additional ways the literature will be useful in your project proposal.

---

### EXHIBIT 5.1 MULTIPLE APPROACHES FOR USING THE LITERATURE IN YOUR PROPOSAL

Although much of this chapter addresses literature review as part of the detailed critique of the literature on your specific topic, the literature also supports other sections of the proposal. For example:

**Problem Statement and Introduction**

As you introduce and make the case for the importance of the clinical problem you want to address, you also describe the background of the problem and document its significance. The literature and other best evidence can be used to help describe both local and broad contexts for the problem. As you note local issues, describe the nature and severity of the specific local problem or system dysfunction to be addressed and relate this to broad national or global issues related to the problem.

**Literature Review and Critique**

This section includes a focus on the systematic literature review you are completing. Describe your literature review methods, including databases searched, key words used, years searched, and inclusion/exclusion criteria. Also, as described in Chapter 6, you will synthesize your findings. This will include organizing and summarizing your literature review, often by themes, then summarizing the strengths and weaknesses of the literature related to your problem of interest.

**Your Project Methods**

In this section, the literature you review will help you gain ideas that can be applied to your project methodology. For example, what data collection methods did you find that were effective and can be applied to your project idea? If you are considering QI methods and policy change, is there enough evidence available that could lead to a clinical policy change?

**Further Literature Use in Your Completed Project**

Once your project is completed, you will return to the literature and place your project findings in the context of the literature. This includes identifying similarities and differences in findings related to your project and others reported in the literature.

## BEGINNING THE LITERATURE REVIEW

A good literature review begins with an understanding of information literacy. *Information literacy* refers to a group of abilities that enable you to discover information, understand how that information was produced, and use it to create new knowledge and/or applications (American Library Association, 2016). In a practical sense, it is a critical thinking activity that involves knowing when information is needed, identifying the type of information needed, accessing the needed information, critically evaluating the information, using the information for a specific purpose, and evaluating the outcomes of the information used (Cheeseman, 2013). Information literacy means you need to locate, read, analyze, and organize the current state of the evidence or science (Galvan & Galvan, 2017). For example, to better understand eating issues experienced by patients with Parkinson disease, you have a responsibility to locate and critique relevant literature as well as to report a synthesis of this information so that you know its worth not only as it applies to your specific project, but its overall value in practice.

Today's technologically oriented world both eases and complicates this literature search process because of the quantity of available information and the rapidly changing nature of that information. Although advanced technologies have made searches much easier to conduct than during the pretechnology days, those same technologies have made searching much more complex because of increased options and the sheer volume of information available.

Although informal reviews have their place, the scholarly, advanced clinical project requires a systematic review. A systematic review progresses in a logical manner, provides rationale for decisions made to guide the search, demonstrates understanding of the literature findings, and is well documented. Enough details of your search should be provided so that others can evaluate your thoroughness and replicate your search. The quality of your review serves as the foundation for your advanced clinical project: If you miss relevant literature, you may repeat work that has already been completed or fail to establish a legitimate case for the significance of your project.

Although it is easy to find information in today's world, it is more challenging to find good information. The review must yield information that can legitimately serve as the basis for your project and withstand scrutiny from the scientific community. Use of a hierarchy of evidence (Polit & Beck, 2020) enables you to identify the strengths/weaknesses of information, and thereby establish its credibility, or lack thereof. Part of being scholarly is addressing the quality of the information you are using so that you assess the credibility of your sources.

## CLARIFY THE TYPE OF REVIEW

There are different types of systematic literature reviews, including formal systematic reviews and scoping reviews of the literature. Both use specific approaches to search for and analyze literature relevant to a given topic, but they have different purposes and aims (Pham et al., 2014). Use the type of literature review that both supports your proposed project and is accepted by your school and project faculty.

Formal systematic reviews and scoping reviews have similarities and differences. Both are systematic, well documented, and yield the information necessary to support your project. The purpose of a formal systematic review is to synthesize the best evidence on a specific research question or problem, while the purpose of a scoping review is to map the existing evidence on a broad topic. Scoping reviews are newer and do not yet have as well-established methodological standards, so their quality and consistency varies. Despite this, both formal systematic and scoping reviews can be used to summarize research activities and find gaps. However, the following are likely:

- Formal systematic reviews will be more focused, while scoping reviews will be broader in nature.
- Formal systematic reviews will provide more depth and quality analysis of research findings, while scoping reviews will simply map what is found.

As you start your clinical project proposal, consider whether a scoping review is adequate to begin your work. Such a review could help establish the extent of current research on a broad topic, determine whether a full systematic review would be useful, summarize research findings, and identify gaps in the current literature (Arksey & O'Malley, 2005). Note that a systematic view of the literature, regardless of the type selected, is essential to your scholarly clinical project and must be completed.

## FORMAL SYSTEMATIC REVIEWS OF THE LITERATURE: THE PROCESS OVERVIEW

The components of a systematic review generate a synthesis, or state-of-the-science summary, of your findings and create a decision trail documenting the process. This chapter discusses how to obtain and critique the literature. Synthesizing the literature is addressed in the next chapter.

The first step in the literature review is to gather relevant information with a broad general search of the literature. As you progress in naming and refining your clinical problem, your advanced clinical project will become more focused, as will your continued review of the literature. It is vitally important to recognize the review of literature as an ongoing process, rather than a discrete step that is conducted and marked off your to-do list, because as your project progresses you will learn about additional concepts and have more precise information to search. Also, the literature can change rapidly, and you must always be working with the most up-to-date information possible.

## THE LITERATURE SEARCH: OBTAINING EVIDENCE

There is an art to searching for and obtaining appropriate literature and this process involves multiple phases. In the early phases of the literature review, the goal is to fine-tune your problem statement. As previously discussed, the problem statement provides a succinct statement of the issue or topic of interest and provides the information needed to further refine your literature search. Early in the process, you will have to make important decisions regarding the search. These decisions relate to databases, key words, inclusion/exclusion criteria, practical/methodological screens, and primary/secondary sources.

### Databases

An initial decision is deciding which databases to search. In early search phases, go beyond the nursing literature to identify how other disciplines are using your topic-of-interest concepts. At minimum, begin the search using PubMed, Cumulative Index to Nursing and Allied Health Literature (CINAHL), Education Resources Information Center (ERIC), and Google Scholar. Keep track of the search terms you use as you search the literature, as well as the number of sources that result from each successive search. Consider whether you need to supplement your electronic database search with additional strategies, such as reviews of tables of contents from professional journals or reviews of the reference lists of articles previously found, to address your project purpose. This is especially useful in early stages to identify how others are naming and framing selected problems. Also, keep a decision trail outlining your process, as further discussed later in this chapter.

### Key Words

In addition to determining the databases to search, the key words you will enter to search the databases need to be determined. This determination begins by listing the key words that come to mind related to the concept; also consider the key words used in relevant articles to help establish the initial boundaries of your topic. The search terms that are preprogramed into the specific databases you are using as a means of organizing content in that particular system also need to be considered. Finally, be sure to use the search engine's ability to combine searches. For example, combining a search for the words *ethics* and *decisions* with the word *or* will broaden the search to articles about ethics and articles about decisions; combining those two words with *and* will limit the search to only those articles that pertain to both ethics and decisions.

### Inclusion/Exclusion Criteria

Next, you need to add further structure to your review. How will you further structure your search if your search provides excessive or irrelevant resources? One benefit of problem statements and purpose statements is that they help identify and clarify the project's scope and limits. For example, if you are reviewing best evidence on pain-management protocols, you will likely need to clarify what patient groups this includes. Chronic pain management with dementia patients has a different context than pain management for those with acute back injuries, so noting the inclusion and exclusion criteria for the search is necessary. *Inclusion criteria* indicate what will be included in the search, and *exclusion criteria* refer to what will be omitted. These concepts are similar to "practical screens," which are discussed further in the next section. Note that in initial stages of the review it may be useful to consider the similarities and differences in how related topics are covered.

Inclusion and exclusion criteria can also be used to keep your project and the literature you find consistent with one another. For example, if your project has to do with a cardiac procedure protocol in an urban hospital intensive care unit, you may want to exclude protocols you find from step down units or rural hospitals. While it is important that the references you use fit your project context and are relevant to your topic, it is also true that a broader search of the literature can sometimes yield new ideas and solutions not previously considered for different contexts. Be sure your review of literature findings fits your topic and context and be sure to explicitly note where ideas from other contexts are being introduced.

### Practical/Methodological Screens

Both practical and methodological screens help frame the topic. *Practical screen* refers to naming the types of references to be included. These practical screen criteria could include, for example, the databases of the disciplines to be considered, publication years to include, and language options (most often limited to English-language articles only). Identifying terms that you will be studying, as well as those terms you are not studying, helps avoid comparing apples to oranges. *Methodological screens* refer to those criteria that clarify the level of study or quality of evidence you are seeking (Fink, 2020). For example, your review might note that only articles that are based on data will be included.

### Primary/Secondary Sources

As you begin to find helpful references, you will make decisions about primary and secondary sources. Recall that primary references contain content written by the original author, while with a secondary source someone else (the secondary source) is reporting on the original author's work (American Psychological Association [APA], 2020). Primary sources are generally recommended in scholarly work because the information comes directly from the person who originally presented it, which eliminates issues of interpretation error or possible bias by another (secondary) author. However, secondary sources can also offer helpful information. For example, often they report on multiple other sources at one time and in one place. So, while primary sources are generally preferred, your review of literature may contain both primary and secondary sources, depending on your topic and your graduate program guidelines.

If you are new to the process, a successful literature search will be facilitated by working with a more experienced searcher, such as a librarian and/or a content expert. The best searches are conducted by people who know both the mechanics of literature searches and the content area. Also, learn from the experience of DNP students who have preceded you in this process. Their advice is presented in the Advice From DNP Students box.

> **ADVICE FROM DNP STUDENTS**
>
> **Literature Review**
>
> Use multiple search engines to get started.
>
> - Initially, keep going back to the literature and immerse yourself in multiple search engines.
> - Spend time with a librarian.
>
> Avoid getting lost in the literature.
>
> - Keep returning to your purpose statement and asking whether this literature—from both formal and informal sources—is related.
> - Know what you are looking for and, if you get lost, go back to your purpose statement.

## CHALLENGES/FACILITATORS TO GAINING THE EVIDENCE

Various challenges may arise when searching the literature. These relate to lack of literature, trouble accessing quality references, and difficulty keeping track of the literature obtained.

### What if You Cannot Find Research/Literature Evidence?

Sometimes even the most systematic search yields no results and this may cause you to draw one of several conclusions. The first possibility is that no evidence currently exists, in which case your advanced clinical project needs to address this situation. The other possibility is that evidence exists but, to date, you have failed to find it. Perhaps you have not yet used the key terms or databases that will lead to the information you need. Optional approaches in this case include expanding your search to databases from other disciplines, stepping back and using different or broader search terms, or seeking consultation with an expert.

Another possibility is that the evidence that exists is not found in the literature per se. In this case, it is important to consider what other types of documents and resources could be counted as evidence. For example, national healthcare professional organizations often serve as clearinghouses and resources for the best evidence. Professional organization websites, such as that of the Alzheimer's Association or the American Diabetes Association, typically provide extensive evidence-based resources that supplement the more traditional review of the literature.

### What if Accessing or Obtaining the Evidence Is Problematic?

Another potential obstacle is that, although you find reference titles that sound worthwhile, the articles are not available to you locally or cost too much to borrow elsewhere. This is a good time to seek the help of a more experienced literature searcher or librarian and, if the desired literature still cannot be accessed, you have a responsibility to note these types of issues and limitations in your proposal.

### What if You Have Trouble Keeping Track of the Search Process?

In addition to saving your literature searches, be sure to keep a decision trail that enables you to reconstruct the decisions made during the search and the rationale that guided the search process. A decision trail is an objective accounting of the processes used in completing the search. This provides a type of accountability in the steps you have taken to ensure a comprehensive search and to provide enough detail so that others could replicate your search.

For example, if your interest is in nursing ethics, how many articles did you find after searching the word *ethics*? What did you find when you then searched the combined words *nursing ethics*? Are you more interested in ethical decision-making in nursing, rather than nursing ethics in general? Were the results different when you used *ethical decision-making*? How many articles did you find for this search phrase and how many of those were relevant to your topic? Did you refine the search further and, if so, using what new key words and why? Now consider the fact that these questions are answered in a very short period of time and the quantity of findings and subsequent decisions grows exponentially. As noted, you will need to determine a system by which you keep track of all these decisions and information.

This concept also extends to what databases were chosen for the search and what rationale led to these decisions. A beginning strategy is to save every search you make, such that you have a record of the terms and search engines used, as well as the search results. Additional notes in the form of a decision trail will remind you at a later time why you made the decisions reflected in your searches. Again, these documents will be important as you summarize in your proposal the systematic approach you used in reviewing the literature. A basic tip is not to trust your memory; rather, document every step and decision in real time.

The following are components that should be included in summarizing the process used for your systematic review. You decision trail should clearly describe

- the databases that you searched;
- search terms and search strategies used, including a summary of search trail/phrases that led you to the articles reviewed;
- the number of articles produced by each separate search, including the number that were relevant to your specific topic;
- inclusion/exclusion criteria (i.e., specific criteria for this review such as literature time frames to consider and populations to consider); and
- the practical/methodological screens considered.

## READING AND CRITIQUING THE EVIDENCE

Once your search is over and you have obtained articles, your activities shift from information seeking to information reading and critiquing. The term *reading* can be misleading in that the process involves much more than just reading. Recall the vast amounts of information available today. This quantity of information requires efficient methods by which to organize, store, and evaluate the merit (or lack thereof) of information obtained.

### To Help in Reading

Use active reading to narrow the field. First, read the abstract and preview the article and then use questions to further consider while reading—questions about studies/findings: who, what, how big/little, where/how outcomes were gained. As you read, consider the following approaches regarding how the article helps you

- identify common themes in the literature,
- clarify interesting points or irritating questions,
- organize/confirm thoughts on a topic,
- consider the feasibility of your project, and
- appraise the worth of your project.

### To Help in Evaluating the Quality of the Evidence

Step three of Melnyk and Fineout-Overholt's (2023) seven steps of evidence-based practice is to critically appraise the evidence. Rapid critical appraisal (RCA) checklists are used to determine whether a study is a "keeper" by evaluating the study's validity, reliability, and helpfulness in respect to the issue being addressed. Evaluate, appraise, and critique the evidence does not mean only criticize the evidence; rather, you must determine its strengths and weaknesses and recognize both as you determine the quality of that evidence and its value to your own work. Basically, the stronger the validity, reliability, and applicability to the topic you're working on, the better the quality of the evidence.

In addition to RCAs, hierarchies of evidence have been developed to help determine the quality and strength of evidence. It is important to identify which hierarchy you are using and to provide a sound rationale for that decision, and then use that hierarchy consistently throughout your advanced clinical project. For example, Polit and Beck (2020) use a seven-level hierarchy ranging from level I (systematic review of RCTs) as the strongest and best evidence, to level VII (opinions of authorities and/or case reports) as the weakest evidence. Both Polit and Beck (2020) and Melnyk and Fineout-Overholt (2023) suggest that the best hierarchy to use depends on the clinical question being asked.

Although RCAs and hierarchies vary, the fundamentals of their appraisal systems are consistent in that studies with the strongest reliability and validity produce the strongest evidence. Other resources are available to determine the quality of other data sources you might encounter in your search. For example, if you have found practice guidelines as part of your evidence search, then you might consider evaluating the guidelines according to the Appraisal of Guidelines for Research and Evaluations II (AGREE; www.agreetrust.org/wp-content/uploads/2013/06/AGREE_II_Users_Manual_and_23-item_Instrument_ENGLISH.pdf). AGREE provides a mechanism for evaluating the quality of existing guidelines, as well as a method for developing strong guidelines.

If your search yields a systematic review or meta-analysis, then you should determine whether it meets the Preferred Reporting Items for Systematic Reviews and Meta-Analyses (PRISMA; www.prisma-statement.org) criteria. PRISMA identifies a minimum set of items that need to be addressed to ensure complete reporting of these types of research activities. As with AGREE, PRISMA provides not only a mechanism for evaluating the quality of evidence found but, in case the rest of your project takes this direction, guidelines for developing and reporting quality work as well.

Remember the basic premise mentioned earlier: "Reading" does not mean just reading; it also means evaluating and critiquing the quality of what you are reading. Keep in mind that there are a variety of tools, such as RCAs, hierarchies, AGREE, and PRISMA, to help you evaluate the quality of the evidence you find. Also, remember that as you conduct this process on each individual piece of evidence you collect, you will also need to appraise the quality of the evidence as a whole, too.

## THE EVIDENCE SUMMARY: ORGANIZING THE LITERATURE REVIEW FINDINGS

As evidence is identified, obtained, read, and critiqued, you will need a mechanism by which to organize all of your information. There are several options, and you will likely need to use more than one of them.

### Archiving and Cataloguing

You will need an organized and competent system for keeping track of the evidence you find. At the very least this should consist of an electronic system, either a commercial application (EndNote, OneNote) or developing your own system using a program such as Excel. These resources provide the opportunity to easily record the references you find and highlight details of the content therein.

### Reference Matrix

The more robust approach to organizing evidence is to use a reference matrix, which may be called by various names, such as bibliography table or summary matrix. A reference matrix is more than just a list of references; rather, it includes content that helps to organize your findings, gain an overview of what you found, and provide a quick summary of what you gained (Galvan & Galvan, 2017). This matrix serves several purposes. First, it helps to organize the growing number of individual articles and evidence you find on your advanced clinical project topic. Second, it provides a beginning synthesis of the literature as a whole, which will be your next step in the process. Third, it also provides the context for how your project can help extend the knowledge/literature on this topic. Paragraphs summarizing and synthesizing the findings that emerge from your matrix are then easily organized into your project proposal. The matrix itself may become an appendix in your proposal. Finally, the matrix serves as a quick snapshot summary of the evidence gathered and an easy communication tool for your team members to use.

### Reference Matrix Format

The reference matrix is generally created in a table format with a row for each piece of evidence (i.e., each research article) and various columns for different information about each piece of evidence. All matrices will include standard information, such as the full article citation, but the remaining columns are guided by the needs of your particular advanced clinical project. You may include, for example, the level of evidence in one column, the methods used in another, and then place the population, the setting, strengths, and weaknesses each in a column of their own. Although you are free to create your own headings for columns in your matrix/table, you will have to include key components. For example, columns or components for the table that are often important to your project include key terms/concepts, definitions, research study methods, critique of the study, and summary of study findings. At a minimum, a reference matrix listing the strengths and weaknesses of each article is needed in your archiving/cataloguing system. Exhibit 5.2 provides an example of headings used in a literature matrix.

The reference matrix can be created using various tools, but common tools include Microsoft Word and Excel. Sometimes a strategy that begins with Excel and then copies and pastes to Word provides advantages. Although creating this matrix may appear to be an extra step at this point in your project, in the long run it will make the critique and synthesis of the literature much easier. Also, recall that the literature is constantly being updated. You will have to consider this a work in progress as you find additional resources to add.

### Final Touches to the Reference Matrix

As you finalize your matrix and prepare to write up your findings from the literature, you may ask whether yours is a reasonable matrix. Consider addressing the following questions:

- How much literature is enough?
- Have you started with a broad approach to the topic and then narrowed your topic adequately to gain the detail of a specific component?
- Have you searched at least one database beyond traditional discipline (nursing) literature?
- Are you getting saturation from the references you are finding (i.e., no new ideas are emerging from articles)?
- Have you considered whether there are classic references to include (i.e., those included in most other reference lists that can provide some historical perspective)?

| EXHIBIT 5.2 SAMPLE REFERENCE MATRIX HEADINGS | | | | | |
|---|---|---|---|---|---|
| Citation | Participants/Setting | Purpose, Background | Methods/Design and Limitations—Hierarchical Level | Findings Summary, Strengths/Weakness | Applicability to Own Project |
|  |  |  |  |  |  |

## Documenting Sources

Documenting sources and the reference format you use are considered parts of written scholarly communication. The format used in the *Publication Manual of the American Psychological Association,* Seventh Edition (APA, 2020) is the one most often used in the nursing profession to ensure that scholarly references are provided in an accessible format. Recording a citation correctly initially saves lots of problems and time down the road; therefore, plan to summarize article notes (in your reference matrix) in a format that can be cited.

## LITERATURE REVIEW TIPS FOR GETTING STARTED

- Focus your literature search by connecting two or more words with *and*.
- Use both nursing and nonnursing search engines.
- Do not rely on memory; rather, take good notes about your search, including search engines used, key words searched, inclusion/exclusion criteria applied, number of articles produced from the search, and the reasons articles were eliminated.
- Briefly scan abstracts to determine whether there is a possible fit with your project before committing to reading full articles.
- Document reference citations in the moment and confirm their accuracy.
- Prepare your reference matrix. Gain guidance from resources such as PRISMA.

### PRACTICE SCHOLARSHIP APPLICATIONS

Consider your competency documentation plans. How will your project address select American Association of Colleges of Nursing (AACN) *Essentials* (2021)? Consider additions to your project notebook as you complete the following.

- *Concepts to competence*: Think about your knowledge of literature searches. What process did you establish to maintain a current and accurate decision trail of your literature search and why did it work? What format best presents your reference matrix content, and why is it the most effective format?
- *Essentials*: Review the competencies for the three *Essentials* domains Informatics and Healthcare Technologies, Scholarship for the Nursing Practice, and Knowledge for Nursing Practice. Reflect on how they relate to your review of the literature.
- *Project notebook*: Include a one-page reflective paper that summarizes your plans for a reference matrix and decision trail. Are you finding that the evidence is strong enough to provide support for your project idea? Is the evidence leading you to change your project idea? Once you are ready, include your full reference matrix (or at least sample pages).

## SUMMARY AND KEY POINTS

Completing a systematic literature review as part of your clinical project is a key component of clinical scholarship. In addition, part of being scholarly is addressing the quality of the information you are using and using credible resources. The systematic literature review and reference matrix provide a beginning point to discuss the credibility of resources/references. Points to recall from this chapter include the following:

- The review of literature provides a basis for further proposal work.
- *Information literacy* consists of finding and understanding existing information and then using it to create new knowledge.
- The goal of the review of literature is to search for and obtain evidence, review and critique the evidence, and then generate an evidence summary.
- Key considerations when obtaining evidence are databases, key words, inclusion/exclusion criteria, practice/methodological screens, and primary/secondary sources.
- Challenges to the evidence search might include trouble finding, accessing, and tracking evidence.
- Summarize the process of searching for evidence in a decision trail.
- Read the evidence that was found, including a critique of both strengths and limitations.
- Read the literature to understand its worth to practice and to your project. Begin to identify common themes in the literature.
- Organize and update the literature review findings, which are essential elements of an efficient process and a well-supported clinical project, in reference matrix format.

## WEBSITES FOR FURTHER REVIEW

Finding current information in relevant and trustworthy online resources can be a challenge. Try the following links for additional information and examples on hierarchies of evidence and guidelines for critiquing articles.

The following resources provide additional content about systematic reviews and examples of levels or hierarchies of evidence:

- *The Cochrane Consumer Network*:

    https://consumers.cochrane.org/cochrane-and-systematic-reviews#systematic:

    https://consumers.cochrane.org/cochrane-and-systematic-reviews#levels

There are also numerous guides that can be used to critique articles. Consider the following as you look for one that you find thorough and user friendly:

- *American Nurses Association, Framework for How to Read and Critique a Research Study*: www.nursingworld.org/~4afdfd/globalassets/practiceandpolicy/innovation--evidence/framework-for-how-to-read-and-critique-a-research-study.pdf
- *Open Michigan, Topic 08—Article Critique*: https://open.umich.edu/documents/nursing/topic-08-article-critique
- *California State University—Long Beach*: https://home.csulb.edu/~arezaei/ETEC551/critique-guide.htm

## NEXT CHAPTER UP

Chapter 6 is about synthesizing the literature review. After completing your reference matrix, the next step is to synthesize this literature into a document that summarizes the overall state of the literature relevant to your problem. This provides you with an opportunity to identify strengths and gaps in the literature on your topic, as well as a possible solution to your problem. The conclusions you draw during the literature review help connect the problem statement to your project purpose statement.

### ONLINE/CLASSROOM DISCUSSION

In discussions with your colleagues, share responses to the following:

- Share with your colleagues one concept essential to your clinical project literature review. What question is guiding your beginning literature search? As you begin your literature search what seems to be the strength(s) of the evidence? Have you had challenges, such as needing to revise your search strategies?
- What suggestions do you have for colleagues as they share their plans? What recommendations can you share with select classmates in their respective literature searches and to help them best find the information they seek?

## LEARNING ACTIVITIES

### To-Do List

1. Work on the decision trail for your systematic literature review. As you progress with your systematic literature review, confirm that you are on track with
   - search terms and strategies described, including specific databases;
   - summary of search trail/phrases that led you to include the articles reviewed;
   - inclusion/exclusion criteria noted (i.e., specific criteria for this review such as literature time frames to consider, populations to consider);
   - practical/methodological screens considered; and
   - primary/secondary sources.
2. Work on your reference matrix. To organize, choose categories that help you best capture information for your synthesis. Include the following, for example:
   - citation
   - participants/setting
   - purpose, background
   - methods/design
   - findings
   - summary of strengths/weakness
   - applicability to your own project

_____

_____

_____

_____

_____

_____

_____

## REFERENCES

American Library Association. (2016). *Framework for information literacy for higher education.* http://www.ala.org/acrl/standards/ilframework

American Psychological Association. (2020). *Publication manual of the American Psychological Association* (7th ed.).

Arksey, H., & O'Malley, L. (2005). Scoping studies: Towards a methodological framework. *International Journal of Social Research Methodological, 8*(1), 19–32. https://doi.org/10.1080/1364557032000119616

Cheeseman, S. E. (2013). Information literacy: Foundation for evidence-based practice. *Neonatal Network, 32*(2), 127–131. https://doi.org/10.1891/0730-0832.32.2.127

Fink, A. (2020). *Conducting research literature reviews: From the internet to paper* (5th ed.). Sage.

Galvan, J. L., & Galvan, M. C. (2017). *Writing literature reviews: A guide for students of the social and behavioural sciences* (7th ed.). Routledge.

Melnyk, B. M., & Fineout-Overholt, E. (2023). *Evidence-based practice in nursing & healthcare: A guide to best practice* (5th ed.). Wolters Kluwer/Lippincott Williams & Wilkins.

Pham, M., Rajic, A., Greig, J., Sargeant, J., Papadopoulos, A., & McEwen, S. (2014). A scoping review of scoping reviews: Advancing the approach and enhancing the consistency. *Research Synthesis Methods, 5*(4), 371–385. https://doi.org/10.1002/jrsm.1123

Polit, D., & Beck, C. T. (2020). *Nursing research generating and assessing evidence for nursing practice* (11th ed.). Lippincott Williams & Wilkins.

# 6. Synthesizing Best Evidence and Literature Review

## INITIAL THOUGHT

"What does literature synthesis mean? Are you sure I can't just describe the evidence article by article?"

## CHAPTER CONTENT

- Reflective Questions
- Quality Improvement Alert
- Creating the Literature Synthesis
  - Begin by Reviewing Your Reference Matrix
  - Move From Individual Article Description to Synthesis and Critique of Matrix Articles
  - Reflect on the Reference Matrix Findings as a Whole
- Organize the Synthesis Summary Statements
- Prewriting the Synthesis
- Moving to the Finished Literature Synthesis
  - Write the Introductory Section to the Literature Synthesis
  - Include the Systematic Literature Review Methods
  - Include Introductory Overview and Summary Statements
  - Consider Further Uses for the Literature Synthesis
- Finishing-Up Checklist for Literature Synthesis
- Relating the Literature Synthesis to the Concept of "Translating" Evidence
- Literature Synthesis Tips to Consider
- Practice Scholarship Applications
- Summary and Key Points
- Websites for Further Review
  - Interprofessional Synthesis Examples
  - Guides for Synthesis Reviews
- Next Chapter Up
- Online/Classroom Discussion
- Learning Activities
  - To-Do List

## REFLECTIVE QUESTIONS

In Chapter 5, you learned about strategies for completing a systematic literature review, including determining the quality of the information you gathered. This chapter takes you through the next step of synthesizing the literature review. The following reflective questions organize learning for this chapter. With which of the following are you most confident?

- What should you do to make the relevant references you found in the literature helpful to your project?
- What does it mean to synthesize the literature?
- What does it mean to identify themes from the literature review?
- Why is the evidence/literature synthesis important to your project?

Use the Practice Scholarship Applications (at the end of this chapter) to help document your learning from concept to competency, including the relevant American Association of Colleges of Nursing (AACN) *Essentials* (2021).

## QUALITY IMPROVEMENT ALERT

Synthesizing the literature pulls together all of the relevant articles/sources you found so that, as a whole, it provides the context and the rationale for your quality improvement (QI) project.

Synthesis of best evidence provides a resource for making evidence easily accessible. Rather than a stack of journal articles, the synthesis is a coherent story of what is known and not known about a particular study area. Although large national study groups convene to develop syntheses on major topics of importance, there is also value in smaller scale syntheses in new study areas, as it enables you to take the references found in your systematic literature review and integrate them into a cohesive summary of your overall findings.

Synthesizing is a step that is additive to the literature review. Synthesis is about describing similarities and differences in articles and drawing conclusions about the literature as a whole, rather than each article individually. It provides the big picture of what research is available (and not available) and its overall quality. It not only incorporates the critique of studies reviewed, but also adds integration, or synthesis, of the results. It involves identifying the strengths and weaknesses of the systematic literature review. Rather than cataloguing, for example, by year of the article, the synthesis provides an easily accessible summary of what is known and not known about your topic from the literature overall.

For example, your colleague has an interest in complementary health approaches for pain management and has reviewed the literature on yoga as a strategy to support pain management. Your colleague was surprised at the variety of ways yoga was defined and the variety of pain-related diagnoses for which yoga was used. Even after creating a matrix of studies on yoga for pain management, they realized that more analysis and a summary of the big picture of the research/evidence on the topic was required. Because of the variation in concept definitions and populations, it was important that your colleague identify similarities and differences so that they could be sure they were comparing similar approaches, or at least clarifying the differences in the types of yoga and the variability in the populations in which it was used. This was done in addition to determining the strengths of the evidence for your colleague's matrix studies.

Just as your hypothetical colleague in the aforementioned example, even after creating your matrix of individual articles, you will need to further analyze and synthesize the big picture of the literature to better understand and convey your topic to others. You need to use the evidence to frame your chosen problem and to identify solutions/strategies that others have used. Your proposal synthesis will include a summary and analysis of findings from the literature search.

Although the introductory section of your proposal uses literature to describe your problem and related issues, this specific literature review section addresses the more detailed systematic review of the literature: You take each article or piece of evidence placed in the reference matrix (as discussed in Chapter 5) and, after comparing and contrasting that evidence, draw conclusions about the findings and the quality of those overall findings. This chapter addresses how to synthesize, or craft, the big picture of the literature review.

## CREATING THE LITERATURE SYNTHESIS

Synthesizing the literature involves moving from a critique of individual articles to describing and commenting on the findings as a whole. Synthesizing adds to the individual article summaries, taking the project to the next level and creating information sharing in a new way via the pulled-together resources (Galvan, 2017). Synthesizing involves

- taking separate articles and blending them into a synthesis of the overall topic to help better understand the state of the evidence related to your problem;
- showing the coherent flow of evidence of the specific literature reviewed, including descriptions of the important concepts/themes and how they fit together into a cohesive whole; and
- sharing a meaningful interpretation, synthesis, and report on the combined literature findings.

Your synthesis will provide a description of the current body of knowledge in your clinical area. It can help make a case of the need for, or the merits and value of, your proposed clinical project. Presenting this synthesis in a logical way with these steps also makes the review more easily accessible to others.

### Begin by Reviewing Your Reference Matrix

The matrix has helped you organize information from your literature review and now helps with easy retrieval and flexible use of your review (Garrard, 2020). To begin the written literature synthesis, you will return to your completed reference matrix. Recall that in your matrix, you have summarized and critiqued the individual studies. Now you are taking what you found in individual articles and describing/analyzing that content as a whole.

Begin by reviewing and critiquing your reference matrix and making sure that it is finalized and ready for synthesis. Check to see whether the following components are complete in your reference matrix:

- References are appropriate, useful, accurately documented, and come from respected publications.
- Your findings are clearly identified from research and other evidence-based sources.
- The summary of each article is relevant, clear, and accurate.
- A strong critique of each reported study is provided.
- Unique or interesting points from each article are noted.

### Move From Individual Article Description to Synthesis and Critique of Matrix Articles

Typically, the first draft of a project's literature review tends to be a compilation of descriptive paragraphs about each individual study reviewed. This is problematic in that the draft is missing (a) the critique of each study and (b) the synthesis of the combined study findings. For example, if your literature review is similar to the following hypothetical project, then you have not yet synthesized the literature:

- Author 1 conducted a correlational study on stress with 50 participants and found frequent comments about crisis and specific relationships to anxiety.
- Author 2's descriptive study looked at anxiety. She interviewed 15 participants and found that subjects related anxiety to stress.

- Author 3 conducted a qualitative study with 10 participants experiencing crisis and found themes of stress and anxiety.

If, in contrast, you have focused more on the following format, then you are on the right track to creating a literature synthesis from these three articles:

- Several studies (Author 1, Author 2, and Author 3) have found that there is a relationship among anxiety, stress, and crisis. Although two of the studies (Author 2 and Author 3) were qualitative in nature and used appropriately small samples, all three support the nature of the concept relationships and need for further study.

## Reflect on the Reference Matrix Findings as a Whole

Now that you have considered what a synthesis of several articles looks like, you are ready to move forward to a larger synthesis of your full reference matrix. As noted previously, you will synthesize your matrix via summaries of content and study methods. Synthesizing the literature does not mean just recounting the references via random listing. It focuses on a summary or synthesis of the big picture of the references reviewed, usually by themes or shared subjects. When summarizing and synthesizing your big-picture review of the literature, the following additional questions and phrases may help you synthesize your literature review in an organized manner (i.e., as you look for themes, strengths, weaknesses, or gaps in current evidence):

- What summary statements can you make about the level of evidence from the various studies/reports and the findings associated with them?
- How much variation was there and how was your concept defined/considered/delivered across the studies/reports?
- How much variation was there in the outcome(s) studied across the studies/reports?
- Was there variation in methods used and, if so, how much?
- What findings are supported by more than one study/report?
- What findings are supported by just one study, but are compelling? Why are they compelling?
- What findings are inconsistent across the studies/reports?
- What findings are outright contradictory across the studies/reports?
- What further questions do you still need to address (Fink, 2019; Garrard, 2020)?

Do not become overwhelmed by the number of articles you need to synthesize. These prompts will help you begin to think about how to group together different articles with related content.

## ORGANIZE THE SYNTHESIS SUMMARY STATEMENTS

Approaches to organizing and synthesizing the literature review include grouping the important themes found in your review, identifying strengths and gaps of the overall literature, identifying variations in concept definitions or populations found in the literature, and noting variations in the quality of the different studies. These findings from the literature then have the potential to be used as headings to help guide the reader through the literature synthesis section. Note that these prompts help you consider the following ways to organize your literature synthesis:

- *Important themes*: This involves identifying each of the main/relevant concepts/themes and then providing a descriptor or definition from the literature. If there are differences in how the term is described, then note this so as to avoid comparing apples to oranges. For example, if "support group" is your topic of interest, are you reviewing online or face-to-face groups (or both)? If both, you will organize findings so that this is reflected.

- *Literature strengths and gaps*: Summarize the strengths of the literature, and then describe gaps or areas with limited research. Summarize the commonalities and the differences of studies within each theme. Add a final summary noting the overall themes and strengths/weaknesses of the literature in describing your problem of interest. If additional themes emerge from your references, the approach (noted earlier) can be completed for each theme.

- *Variations in concept definitions or populations*: In the introductory example, the definitions of yoga and the populations using yoga were quite diverse. Multiple studies were noted using varied concept definitions and treatment definitions that could not be used easily for outcome comparisons. Organizing your synthesis by grouping together varied definitions that are similar can be a useful approach. This will be an important point to convey in your synthesis summary, noting that the current literature (with diverse definitions and approaches for the same concepts) makes comparisons and generalizations challenging.

- *Variation in methods quality*: Also consider methodological themes informing the quality of the findings as a way to organize the literature synthesis. For example, randomized controlled studies with large samples provide very strong evidence compared with small descriptive studies. Critique your reference matrix and

## EXHIBIT 6.1 LONG-TERM CARE COMMUNICATION: SUMMARY OF LITERATURE REVIEW SYNTHESIS

**Linda Kroeger, DNP**

*Methods*

A systematic literature review was conducted. Databases searched include PubMed, Cumulative Index of Nursing and Allied Health Literature (CINAHL), and Google Scholar. The keywords are *nursing home*, *long-term care*, *communication*, *telephone medicine*, *quality improvement*, and *nurse–physician relations*. The literature review included research studies and articles from 1997 to 2011 and was limited to healthcare. Articles were excluded if they were not related to healthcare professionals or communication. References from key articles were also retrieved and reviewed. The review revealed that one group of researchers from Duke Medical Center did extensive work on this topic. Author searches were done on each member of this group. The following themes organized the literature review: an overview of communication issues, barriers to effective communication, improving telephone communication in LTC, and liability issues.

*Literature Synthesis Review Summary*

Many studies look specifically at telephone communication between LTC nurses and physicians. These studies addressed barriers to communication, the importance of communication, and methods to improve communication. The studies also described how structured communication can improve the quality of care or how poor communication can lead to error and liability for the provider and facility. Many of these studies have addressed after-hours phone calls in the setting of Veterans Affairs nursing homes and/or physician training programs. These facilities have physicians on site during daytime hours. The literature does not address phone calls to physicians during daytime business hours. For LTC facilities and physicians without daytime on-site coverage, multiple phone calls are disruptive to the office staff and, unless it is an emergency, the LTC nurse often waits long periods to return a call. Many of the studies evaluated the interventions aimed at improving physician skills with telephone communication. Few studies focused on interventions to improve nursing skills with telephone communication. No research looked at RN and LPN roles in communicating with the physician even though the LPN is rapidly becoming the primary nurse caregiver in the LTC setting. Several studies demonstrated that relatively brief clinical educational programs were effective in teaching both RNs and physicians how to better communicate clinical information to other professionals.

*Note*: This example consists of excerpts only and does not constitute a full literature synthesis, but rather a summary of a literature synthesis. The full synthesis would include in-text citations for each article referenced.

---

summarize what was found. Questions that you used in critiquing your matrix findings can assist with your write-up as well.

Note that Exhibit 6.1 provides an example with a literature synthesis final summary. The themes summarized are broad communication issues, barriers to effective communication, improving telephone communication in LTC, and potential liability issues. In your full synthesis of the literature review, you will also incorporate article summaries, critiques, and citations.

## PREWRITING THE SYNTHESIS

To help you get started writing your literature synthesis, create a basic outline. Outlining your synthesis includes detailing the following:

1. Write an introductory statement to the literature review reminding the reader of the review's purpose and explaining the significance of the concepts to be described.
2. Provide evidence of a current, comprehensive, and synthesized literature review that includes a clear description of literature review search methods (i.e., search engines, key words, and inclusion/exclusion criteria).
3. Once key themes or categories are identified, then outline these with specific references. Some find it helpful to begin write-ups with a PowerPoint summary. The small space for text in each of the PowerPoint slides forces an economy of words and a focus on what is most important in the synthesis.
4. Within headings of each concept or theme from your review, summarize the major approach of the studies referenced in a few sentences.
5. At the end of each major concept/theme discussion, summarize the key points supported. In addition, you will include a written summary statement at the end of the full literature synthesis explaining the knowledge available on your topic as well as the gaps in the literature. You can then finish by discussing conclusions/implications from the literature that support your project approach as a logical next step.

## MOVING TO THE FINISHED LITERATURE SYNTHESIS

### Write the Introductory Section to the Literature Synthesis

Briefly remind the reader why this literature review is important and its purpose (i.e., to enhance/support your project). Include for the readers an introduction that provides a map of what will be covered in the literature review section (Galvan, 2017). Mentioning the section subheadings here, in the same order they are presented in the narrative, is a good way to help readers know what content is to come. Also, state the limits of the review or what will not be covered. For example, this review addresses only adult patients and not children. Recall your purpose for the literature synthesis. Remind the reader what you mean by the terms and why this is an important topic.

### Include the Systematic Literature Review Methods

Begin the literature review section with a summary of the methods used for your systematic review. This must include the primary search strategies, including at a minimum the databases searched, key words or phrases included, and time boundaries of the literature, if any. To document your review methods, go back to your decision trail and list the databases and the key phrases searched.

### Include Introductory Overview and Summary Statements

Recall the benefits of introductory and summary statements. A feature of this literature synthesis is to communicate to others what you have learned; therefore, it is important to make this section especially easy for your readers to follow. This is facilitated by beginning each subsection with an overview of what is to be presented and then summarizing at the end of each subsection exactly what was presented. Although it may seem redundant to you, it helps the reader who is not so intimately familiar with your project to stay on track.

### Consider Further Uses for the Literature Synthesis

Your literature synthesis is important both before and after the project implementation. Although the need exists to understand the status of the literature prior to project development (as a component of the proposal), it is also important to return to the synthesis after the project is completed. As a component of the final project analysis, the synthesis provides a way to tie your work back to the professional literature. This helps to show how your project results are similar or different from the findings that others have gained with similar or related projects. Your published project can then help extend what is known about the topic.

## FINISHING-UP CHECKLIST FOR LITERATURE SYNTHESIS

The following points provide guidance in synthesizing the literature and help confirm that you are on the right track in reviewing and synthesizing the literature specific to your chosen problem. Did you

- use headings to provide visual signals for the reader;
- summarize at the end of each subsection, describing the major themes related to your problem and project purpose, and then discussing how the themes are related;
- minimize the use of direct quotes as excessive quotes slow the reader down, so only the most pertinent or necessary direct quotes should be included;
- read and review for logical presentation and coherence; and
- discuss implications of the literature findings specifically related to your project purpose?

## RELATING THE LITERATURE SYNTHESIS TO THE CONCEPT OF "TRANSLATING" EVIDENCE

Synthesizing the literature relates to translating the evidence. Many terms and models exist to describe this process of translation, including research utilization and knowledge transfer. The common approach of initially synthesizing the evidence exists across terms and models. Different approaches may be used, but important concepts in synthesis include understanding the building blocks of your evidence (ideally, well-crafted studies), organizing that evidence, and then making it available for further evaluation. Challenges and strategies related to integrating knowledge from the literature into practice exist, such as making the vast amount of knowledge into an accessible format and making sure health professionals know that this information exists. Varied models have been developed to assist with that translation (White et al., 2019).

Nurses can translate that evidence, which basically requires synthesizing the available evidence into meaningful, useful protocols and then implementing and evaluating those protocols for utility. For example, with chronic pain/relaxation protocols, search first for strong studies with a tight experimental design. Additional data (if extensive experimental data are not available) can be gleaned from descriptive data and practitioner reports. After gaining the best evidence base, organize this information into protocol format for further testing. Further testing of evidence can be done by implementing and evaluating the protocol.

This chapter has particular relevance for clinical projects that involve evidence summaries. For example, with chronic pain management, one of the top disabling medical problems, there are a variety of medication and nonmedication approaches available. The purpose of a sample project might relate to determining what nondrug-related approaches are useful to people with chronic pain. For example, what does the evidence say about relaxation strategies and chronic pain?

Good clinical projects include an evidence-based focus indicating synthesis of the literature. Learning strategies for synthesizing versus cataloguing will serve you well in future projects. Strategies for review and critique of synthesis articles, as noted in Chapter 5, such as Preferred Reporting Items for Systematic Reviews and Meta-Analyses (PRISMA) and Appraisal of Guidelines for Research and Evaluation II (AGREE), provide further guidance for review of synthesis articles.

## LITERATURE SYNTHESIS TIPS TO CONSIDER

The literature synthesis requires combining together content from multiple sources. The following system with a focus on color coding can help:

- Be sure your literature matrix is complete and accurate, and includes columns for key content of interest, such as populations and methods.
- Use color codes on the matrix itself to highlight similar themes within each area: content/findings, populations, and methods. Highlight, for example, all of the methods-related content from each article in yellow, all of the population content from each article in green, and all of the findings from each article in blue.
- Pull information together from the multiple articles that have the same color; for example, write your first synthesis paragraph about methods by pulling together all of the content highlighted in yellow. This will make it easier to synthesize content about the three qualitative, seven descriptive, and three correlational studies that were found, or the 10 quasi-experimental, five randomized controlled trials, and two meta-analyses that were found.
- Review what you have written; if your paragraphs combine content on similar topics from multiple articles you are on the right track, but if each of your paragraphs describe only an individual article, then you need to backtrack and redirect your focus to synthesis.
- Remember to include an introductory overview and summary statements at the beginning and end of each synthesis section.

## SUMMARY AND KEY POINTS

Synthesizing the literature can provide a critical analysis and summary of the existing literature in your clinical area of interest. In developing this synthesis of the best evidence on your topic, you describe the current state of the overall evidence or science. Through identification of the strengths and weaknesses of the overall body of evidence in your problem area, you provide the rationale for your project. You describe the significance of your proposed clinical project proposal and how it will extend the knowledge on this topic. Your conclusions about the literature serve to frame the problem you intend to address and the approach you propose. A good synthesis allows you to move your proposal forward in creating a succinct problem statement and generating a project purpose statement. Points to recall from this chapter include the following:

> **PRACTICE SCHOLARSHIP APPLICATIONS**
>
> Consider your competency documentation plans. How will your project address select *Essentials*? Consider additions to your project notebook as you complete the following.
>
> - *Concepts to competence*: Consider your knowledge about literature synthesis. What themes or topics provided the most useful guidance for organizing and synthesizing your overall literature together? Has the literature synthesize come together to support your clinical project? Why or why not?
> - *Essentials*: Review the advanced level competencies for the two *Essential* domains Scholarship for Nursing Practice and Knowledge for Nursing Practice. Reflect on how they relate to your synthesis of the literature.
> - *Project notebook*: Insert your full literature synthesis (or, at a minimum, a one-page written outline of your review of literature findings). Include your introductory paragraph, overall literature themes, definitions, and methodologies, with supporting literature references included for each. Include your concluding paragraph.

- The literature synthesis moves from critiquing individual articles to describing and critiquing the literature findings as a whole.
- Begin the literature synthesis by reviewing your reference matrix.
- Organize the synthesis summary statements by important themes, literature strengths and gaps, variations in the concept definitions or populations, and/or variations in the methods quality.
- Prewriting the literature synthesis as a basic outline is a helpful way to get started.
- Check your work by confirming that, within each paragraph, you compare multiple references on the given topic, rather than simply describing one study on the topic at a time.

## WEBSITES FOR FURTHER REVIEW

### Interprofessional Synthesis Examples

Examples of syntheses of literature and summaries of next steps can be found in many national reports. Numerous literature syntheses (and practice guidelines) can be found at the Agency for Healthcare Research and Quality (AHRQ). The following URLs provide examples of syntheses on diverse topics, completed by large professional or national organizations. In addition, the National Academy of Sciences (www.nationalacademies.org/) provides reports, including syntheses of the literature. For example, obesity and its complications present a large problem in healthcare. The following national report shows how evidence has been synthesized first on the problem and then on solutions. Potential for further syntheses would exist, for example, on teens, older adults, and other unique populations.

- *Accelerating Progress in Obesity Prevention: Solving the Weight of the Nation*:
  https://nap.nationalacademies.org/hmd/Reports/2012/Accelerating-Progress-in-Obesity-Prevention.aspx
- *AHRQ Evidence-Based Reports*:
  www.ahrq.gov/research/findings/evidence-based-reports/index.html

### Guides for Synthesis Reviews

As noted, guides have been developed to help review the quality of systematic reviews, a large-scale type of synthesis.

- PRISMA:
  www.prisma-statement.org
- AGREE II:
  www.agreetrust.org/wp-content/uploads/2013/06/AGREE_II_Users_Manual_and_23-item_Instrument_ENGLISH.pdf

## NEXT CHAPTER UP

Concepts, theories, and conceptual models provide excellent tools to help organize clinical projects. These concepts, theories, and models provide an organizational framework that establishes the boundaries and conceptual definitions for your project. Chapter 7 addresses frameworks to guide your project.

### ONLINE/CLASSROOM DISCUSSION

In discussions with your colleagues, share feedback with one another on the following:

- Share your introductory paragraphs (or one-page summaries of your syntheses). After considering individual classmates' literature review summaries, what are strengths and weaknesses of the syntheses?

## LEARNING ACTIVITIES

### To-Do List

1. Critique your reference matrix. Make sure it is ready to move to synthesis format. Affirm you have provided
   - a clear description of literature-review methods and project components/processes, and
   - evidence of current, comprehensive literature review documented via your decision trail.

2. Begin the synthesis of your literature review. As you seek themes from your reference matrix, have you
   - considered how much variation there was in how your concept was defined/considered/delivered across the studies/reports;
   - addressed how much variation there was in the outcome(s) studied across the studies/reports;
   - considered what findings were supported by more than one study/report;
   - considered findings that were inconsistent across the studies/reports;
   - thought about findings that were unique, but compelling;
   - considered summary statements you can make about the level of evidence from the various studies/reports and the findings associated with them; and
   - thought about further questions that you still think need to be addressed?

## REFERENCES

Fink, A. (2019). *Conducting research literature reviews: From the internet to paper* (5th ed.). Sage.

Galvan, J. (2017). *Writing literature reviews: A guide for students of the social and behavioural sciences* (7th ed.). Routledge.

Garrard, J. (2020). *Health sciences literature review made easy: The matrix method* (6th ed.). Jones & Bartlett.

White, K., Dudley-Brown, S., & Terhaar, M. (2019). *Translation of evidence into nursing and healthcare* (3rd ed.). Springer Publishing Company.

# 7. Framing the Advanced Clinical Project With Relevant Conceptual Frameworks

## INITIAL THOUGHT

"Don't be wary of using a theory/conceptual model."

## CHAPTER CONTENT

- Reflective Questions
- Quality Improvement Alert
- The Importance of Theories and Conceptual Models
- What It Means to Frame a Project: The Project Triangle
- The Purpose of Concepts
- The Purpose of Frameworks
- Selecting an Appropriate Framework
- Sample Frameworks
- Advice From DNP Students
- Practice Scholarship Applications
- Summary and Key Points
- Websites for Further Review
- Next Chapter Up
- Online/Classroom Discussion
- Learning Activities
  - To-Do List
  - Reflective Prompts
  - Activity

## REFLECTIVE QUESTIONS

In Chapter 6, you learned about synthesizing the best evidence found in your literature review. Now it is time to think about the big picture and what conceptual framework will tie together all of the aspects of your project—the existing literature you have found, the problem you have identified, the project you propose to conduct, and the findings of that project—into a cohesive and organized whole. The following reflective questions organize learning for this chapter. With which of the following are you most confident?

- How do concepts and their definitions help guide a project?
- What is a theory or conceptual framework?
- What does it mean to frame a project?
- Why is this important?
- What is an appropriate framework to use?

Use the Practice Scholarship Applications (at the end of this chapter) to help document your learning from concept to competency, including the relevant American Association of Colleges of Nursing (AACN) *Essentials* (2021).

## QUALITY IMPROVEMENT ALERT

Conceptual models and theories are helpful in organizing all projects. For your quality improvement (QI) project, focus on frameworks as described in this chapter that are specific for guiding QI projects.

## THE IMPORTANCE OF THEORIES AND CONCEPTUAL MODELS

Theories and conceptual models serve as an organizing framework used to guide clinical projects or organize plans for change. The right framework provides organization for proposal writing as well. In Chapters 5 and 6, you learned about finding evidence and synthesizing the relevant literature for your project. That literature helped to focus your problem statement, while at the same time providing its broader context. In this chapter, you will concentrate on placing your clinical project into an appropriate and useful framework.

The need for a framework to guide projects is universal. Consider the prospect of trying to improve healthcare quality in the United States without any direction at all—how would you know where to start and what to do? In 2011, the U.S. Department of Health and Human Services released a framework to guide its work on the National Strategy for Quality Improvement in Health Care (now called the National Quality Strategy [NQS]). Based on the latest evidence and input from a broad range of stakeholders, the NQS identifies three aims for healthcare: better care, affordable care, and healthy people and communities. Further guidance is provided via six priorities: (a) reducing the harm associated with healthcare, (b) engaging people and families in their own care, (c) promoting good communication and coordination of care, (d) promoting effective prevention and treatments, (e) engaging communities to promote health-related best practices, and (f) making quality care affordable. Although still a daunting task, the NQS framework provides broad direction on how to go about improving healthcare.

For the purposes of this text, the terms *theory*, *conceptual framework*, *conceptual model*, and *framework* are used interchangeably. That is not to deny the important historical conversation about distinctions in terminology that has transpired, but what is relevant here is that theories, frameworks, and/or conceptual models can all serve the required purpose of guiding the clinical project. A clinical project of very broad scope may benefit the most from a broad, systems theory or conceptual framework, whereas a project of very limited scope would benefit from a situation-specific theory. Again, *theory*, *conceptual framework*, *conceptual model*, and *framework* are used interchangeably in this text to refer to the guiding framework for your clinical project.

## WHAT IT MEANS TO FRAME A PROJECT: THE PROJECT TRIANGLE

Recall the project triangle, with its points identified as the project's purpose, methods, and outcomes. Building on the aspect of conceptual models as drawings or depictions of a theory, the triangle itself represents a framework for the clinical project, as it connects those points with three straight lines. The lines provide the boundaries for the clinical project and enclose the concepts involved, providing the overall consistency needed for the project. As long as the three lines remain in the shape of a triangle, the framework provides structure and holds the project together in a consistent and cohesive whole. Note that the triangle itself is supported by context and resources, and all of this is bound by an outer circle consisting of best evidence and theories/conceptual models as a guiding framework.

## THE PURPOSE OF CONCEPTS

Concepts refer to select, reality-based entities. They have been described as mental representations or understandings of phenomena of interest (Walker & Avant, 2019). Clear descriptions can help communicate a specific concept and differentiate similar but unique concepts and their relationships. Concepts can be broad general terms or named specifically for your project. They can be concrete or abstract and vary from simple to complex. The context in which the concepts will be applied needs to be conveyed. The process of naming, defining, and operationalizing is considered a component of concept analysis.

In guiding a project, concepts need to be clearly named and defined; they also need to be operationalized. For example, if the concept of interest is alcohol abuse, a clear name and definition is needed. Is it different from excess alcohol intake? What does that mean? Clear communication about these choices is needed, so all team members and other engaged individuals know what the project addresses. Walker and Avant (2019) suggest using the process of concept analysis, through which the defining characteristics as well as the antecedents and consequences of the concept you intend to investigate are clearly and methodically identified. Through this process, you identify a precise theoretical definition of the concept, which is the basis for concept operationalization.

Operationalizing concepts involves linking your named/described concepts to their measurement for your project. How will the concepts be evaluated? For example, if implementing a sleep health promotion protocol in the hospital, how do you name and describe sleep? Is it measured as a patient's perception of quality sleep, perceived hours slept, lack of morning fatigue? Is it measured by staff observation of sleep time? How accurate will the measurement be? For example, if addressing patients' perception of quality sleep, will this be evaluated using yes/no questions, or completing a rating scale? If it is operationalized as staff's perception of patient sleep, will the observer answer a yes/no question or use other means? Different approaches exist but the goal will be for the most reliable and valid measure.

If wondering about a cause/effect with a certain sleep protocol (i.e., no visitors, no phone, and spaced staff interactions), then the protocol concepts may be considered independent variables (the protocol); and the outcome (quality of sleep) as the dependent variable. Concept definitions and any projected relationships need to be clearly named and described to provide a clear guide for your project. What are the concepts of interest in your project? How will you name and define these?

## THE PURPOSE OF FRAMEWORKS

Frameworks serve several important purposes in clinical projects, but those purposes are so fundamental that the use of frameworks is often unconscious and their role unnoticed. Whether explicit or implicit, frameworks are invariably used to guide clinical projects. For example, in the project "What Nurses Need to Know About Sleep Apnea" (Morton, 2012), the theories are not explicitly identified, but clearly, both physiological and learning frameworks were used. Another project, "Applying Lean and Six Sigma to Your Dermatology Practice" (Rice & Haycraft, 2012), explicitly describes how the frameworks of Lean and Six Sigma can be used in practice. More specific purposes of theoretical frameworks as they apply to clinical projects are described.

- *Boundaries*: Theories/conceptual models are abstractions of reality and, as such, they represent real situations in nursing. The framework used to guide a clinical project should provide a foundation for the project and establish the extent of its scope.
- *Structure and relationships*: The framework also provides a structure within the established boundaries by identifying the concepts included in the project and, depending on the framework, how they are related to

one another. In a patient-teaching/-learning project, the appropriate theory/conceptual model includes patients, teaching/learning, and outcomes. It also suggests the relationship among these concepts as, for example, the link between teaching strategies and outcomes will vary for different aged (child or adult) patients.

- *Concept definitions within a framework*: The concepts used within a framework are defined according to their meaning in the context of the theory/conceptual model. Part of your work in choosing a framework involves critiquing its concepts, how they are defined, and how they are related within the framework. Operationalizing, defining, and relating the concepts as they apply to the specific project is essential to providing organization, structure, and efficiency. For example, in a rehabilitation setting dealing with stroke patients with decreased functional abilities, a new evidence-based team protocol is initiated. The intent is to improve patient functional ability. In this simple example, the context and population are described. The conceptual relationship to be studied in this project is the new team protocol (Evidence-Based Guide for Increasing Activity) and its impact on the improved functional abilities of the patients (score on the Functional Independence Measure [FIM]). This conceptual model (protocol impacting outcomes) accomplishes the noted purposes of a framework.

- *Efficiency*: Because the theory/conceptual model provides boundaries and structure, and perhaps even direction, it increases the efficiency of the project. For example, the framework provides common definitions for the concepts so that confusion about terminology is eliminated.

- *Organization*: With the borders, structure, and direction provided, frameworks may offer several other practical benefits. The theory/conceptual model framework, for example, may suggest a means by which to organize a questionnaire and/or provide substantive content for the questions asked.

- *Consistency*: Although theories/conceptual models do provide the previously stated benefits, they also provide a means of tying those individual benefits together into a consistent, cohesive, and comprehensive whole. The framework is the means to achieving consistency among the project purpose, the methods, and the outcomes.

## SELECTING AN APPROPRIATE FRAMEWORK

The most appropriate framework is the one that best fits your clinical project, and that fit is determined by evaluating potential frameworks for a good match. In fact, critiquing potential frameworks is an essential element of selecting an appropriate theory for a project (McEwen & Wills, 2019). Nursing has a strong tradition of dialogue about the appropriate criteria on which to critique theories (Chinn & Kramer, 2019; McEwen & Wills, 2019; Meleis, 2018; Peterson & Bredow, 2020). To guide the clinical project, following are suggested criteria for evaluating the appropriateness of potential theoretical/conceptual model frameworks.

- *Scope*: One criterion for choosing an appropriate framework is how broad or narrow the focus of the framework is and how well that focus fits the scope of your clinical project. If the project focuses on patient education, then a broad theory/conceptual model is too general and the focus of the project is lost. Conversely, a framework with too narrow a focus will potentially omit vital concepts. Consider focusing on the clinical project as you would if looking through a camera lens. If the wide-angle focus is too broad, the patient being taught may be barely identifiable in the picture; conversely, if what is visible through the lens is too narrow, then the patient may be cut out of the picture altogether.

- *Context*: The framework provides the context of the project, and that context must be consistent with the project. If the project has to do with teaching dressing changes at home, then the theory/conceptual model must address that residential context, as teaching a patient to do in-hospital dressing changes where supplies are abundant and patient time is protected, is far different from at-home dressing changes where the supplies may have run out and there are competing demands from work and family.

- *Logic*: The framework used for the project must be logical and make sense. This does not require in-depth testing; it may simply be a matter of whether the framework makes sense in your own experience. For example, does the teaching theory/conceptual model suggest that the most beneficial relationship between the patient and teacher is that they ignore each other? If so, the theory/conceptual model does not make sense. But if the framework suggests that interaction between the patient and teacher is desirable, then it does make sense.

- *Assumptions*: Frameworks are based on assumptions and those assumptions need to be consistent with the clinical project. For example, some education theories/conceptual models may assume that learners are ready and want to learn, whereas other theories do not make that same assumption. So, if the clinical project aims to address the education of newly diagnosed and resistant teenaged patients with diabetes, then the educational theory/conceptual model that assumes the learner is ready to learn would not be appropriate.

- *Usefulness*: There is no reason to consider a framework that is not useful to your work. Therefore, the theory/

conceptual model must at least include the concepts that are inherent in the clinical project, as well as pertinent information about how those concepts are related. Consider, for example, the project of building a house. Before the actual building project begins, a picture (conceptual model) of the house is drawn and serves to keep the project on course throughout the building process.

- *Simplicity*: Although vitally important, the framework itself is not the topic of the project, so it should not be complicated or demand undue time and effort to explain. Rather, the framework should be easy to understand and not detract from the time and focus spent on the project itself. The theory/conceptual model selected plays a vital, but supporting, role in the project.

In addition to the preceding criteria, there are several other aspects of choosing a framework not listed because they have little practical relevance for us and therefore do not need to be given a great deal of attention. For example, choose the framework that best fits your project and do not spend time worrying about whether it is a nursing theory/conceptual model, or one borrowed from another field. Many important theories/conceptual models that guide patient education arise from other fields such as education and psychology, and their practical contributions should not be ignored just because they were not developed within the nursing profession. Similarly, do not worry if your project requires the use of multiple theories/conceptual models. For example, in the case of patient education, it may be important to use not only a cognitive-developmental theory/conceptual model but also a behavioral-learning theory/conceptual model. Similarly, do not be concerned if you find several frameworks, any or several of which would be useful and appropriate for your project. There may not be just one, absolutely right framework; rather, any one of several frameworks might serve your purpose.

## SAMPLE FRAMEWORKS

There are lots of theories and conceptual models that could serve as potential project frameworks. That means there is likely to be at least one framework that will be helpful to your project, but the task of finding the most appropriate framework for the project might be daunting. Remember that the framework is not the focus of the project; its job is to quietly support and guide your project. If there is one obvious theory/conceptual model to serve as a project framework, great. If not, there may be several that would be equally good. Commonly used frameworks include (but are not limited to) QI, physiology, change, teaching/learning, developmental psychology, systems, management, leadership, and social psychology. There are generally numerous options of theories/conceptual models from which to choose, and a good first step is to brainstorm known frameworks that might work for this project. Also, conduct a cursory review of the literature to see what other possible frameworks you find that might fit your project. The objective is not to find the most complicated and obscure theoretical/conceptual model framework, but rather to find a fairly comprehensive list of potential frameworks for your project. Table 7.1 provides suggestions for several different project topics and potentially appropriate theories.

The plan-do-check-act (PDCA) QI theory/conceptual model, for example, could be used to guide the improvement process of a new employee orientation high-fidelity patient simulation learning experience. Initially the staff plans revisions based on feedback from the previous orientation

**TABLE 7.1 SAMPLE PROJECT TOPICS AND THEORIES**

| Project Topic | Potential Theoretical Frameworks |
| --- | --- |
| Quality improvement | PDCA |
| | Six Sigma |
| | Lean |
| | Deming's theory of profound knowledge |
| Change the care delivery system | Systems |
| | Change |
| | Quality improvement |
| | Transformational leadership |
| | Theory of reasoned action |
| Improve treatment of patient pain | Selye's general adaptation syndrome |
| | Gate control theory |
| | Opponent process theory |
| | Motivation–decision model |
| Determining the child's role in care | Psychoanalytic child development |
| | Cognitive child development |
| | Behavioral child development |
| | Social child development |
| Implementing a new program on smoking cessation | Health belief model |
| | Self-efficacy |
| | Motivational theories |
| Research utilization and evidence-based practice | Iowa model |
| | Star model |
| Patient education | Behavioral learning theories |
| | Cognitive theory |
| | Adult learning |

PDCA, plan-do-check-act.

experience. Goals for the simulation experience and the changes needed to meet those goals are explored. Once the plan is set, changes are implemented in the "do" phase of the theory/conceptual model. After implementation, the simulation and outcomes are reevaluated in the check phase. This then leads to the action step of the improvement process cycle as the check analysis is the basis for continued changes and improvements in future, new employee orientation sessions.

Although numerous frameworks can be considered for a project, it is the match between the project and the framework that is important. If multiple potential frameworks emerge, the next step is to determine which theory/conceptual model is the most appropriate for the project. For example, if the project's purpose is to implement a change in care delivery, then potential theories/conceptual models might include systems, change, quality improvement, transformational leadership, or the theory of reasoned action. But, as your purpose statement is refined and becomes more focused, you will identify additional details that determine which theory/conceptual model best fits the specific purpose and scope of your project. For example, if the purpose evolves into focusing on a change in care delivery to improve patient outcomes, then a QI framework might fit best. But, if the purpose evolves into focusing on the role of the nurse in implementing system changes, then perhaps the theory/conceptual model that best matches that purpose will be transformational leadership. If the purpose evolves into focusing on the change process itself, then change theory may be most appropriate.

Do not be afraid to try a new theory or conceptual model as the framework for your project, especially when more than one type of theory/conceptual model might work. For example, many clinical projects are focused on quality improvement, even if they improve quality through a variety of ways such as education or patient care delivery. So, although a more familiar teaching/learning or patient care delivery theory might work well in these cases, a less familiar QI theory/conceptual model might better serve your purpose (either alone, or in conjunction with an educational or care delivery theory). Again, you are looking for a theory/conceptual model that is easy to use and fits your project. A theory/conceptual model that is new to you but not too hard to learn might focus on the QI aspect of your project and be a better fit than other theories. Consider, for example, the plan-do-study-act (PDSA) model to implement and test QI changes—the model truly is as easy as it sounds to apply in practice. Or expand your framework to the model for improvement, which consists of addressing three basic questions (i.e., What is the goal? How will improvement be established? What changes can be made to produce improvement?), followed by the PDSA cycle (New York State Department of Health, 2020). You could take it even a step further and apply an educational theory; for example, within the overall model for improvement. There are lots of options, so do not confine yourself to a predetermined theory that you like and want to make work, but rather find a theory or theories that will support your project.

Once you have reviewed the project topics and theories listed in Table 7.1, think about your own project topic. Identify at least three potential frameworks that might be useful in guiding your work. If you need more ideas and examples, there are several websites that house project titles and abstracts. One such site option is offered by Vanderbilt University (www.readkong.com/page/fullscreen/2021-dnp-projects-vanderbilt-university-school-of-nursing-4554479), where you will find examples such as the following (pp. 37, 48, 53, respectively):

- Koel, who conducted a 2021 project titled, "Smartphone Reference Application: Emergency Ultrasound for Emergency Nurse Practitioner Students," using the Iowa model to guide the project.

- Perry's 2021 project, "Evaluation of Unit-Based Care Team Implementation and Effect on Length of Stay," for which she used the logic model as a guide.

- Taylor used the plan-do-act (PDA) cycle to guide her 2021 project titled, "Identifying Barriers and Potential Solutions to Obtaining a MAT Waiver for Primary Care Providers."

Another good site that identifies many clinical projects is Scholarworks, offered through the University of Massachusetts (www.umass.edu/nursing/research/doctor-nursing-practice-scholarly-projects). There you will find, for example:

- Canfield's 2020 project, "Health Literacy Universal Precautions: A Quality Improvement Project to Promote Effective Use of Clear, Plain Language Communication Within Primary Care," for which she used Lewin's theory of planned change as a guide.

- Ameck used the chronic care model to guide his 2019 project, "Using Smartphone Technology to Enhance Self-Management Support in Adults With Type 2 Diabetes in Primary Care."

- Lunardi, who used cognitive behavioral therapy in her 2020 project, "Improving Insomnia With Digital Cognitive Behavioral Theory in Patients With Diabetes."

Now reflect on the list of three potential theories/conceptual models you created earlier and critique each framework for its fit with the planned purpose statement for your specific project. Keep in mind the project triangle discussed at the beginning of this chapter. Which framework fits best with the three triangle points: purpose, methods, and outcomes? As the purpose and outcomes have become more focused, generally one or maybe two frameworks begin to emerge as the best and most appropriate for guiding your project. If you still have several good choices, one useful approach is to pick the best known theory, as it will serve to support and facilitate the project without demanding undue time or attention.

The box titled Advice From DNP Students provides helpful advice about selecting a framework for your project.

> **ADVICE FROM DNP STUDENTS**
>
> **Selecting a Clinical Framework**
>
> Clearly name and describe your concepts.
>
> - Be sure to name and define concepts clearly. This is more complex than one would think.
> - There is much detail and thought that goes behind what seem to be simple concepts. Enjoy the thought process. Language has to be explicit.
>
> Figure out the importance of the theory/framework.
>
> - Theory is not my strongpoint. Figure out the importance and the role theoretical frameworks have in your proposal.

> **PRACTICE SCHOLARSHIP APPLICATIONS**
>
> Consider your competency documentation plans. How will your project address select *Essentials*? Consider additions to your project notebook as you complete the following items:
>
> - *Concepts to competence*: Think about your knowledge of concepts and theories/conceptual models. What have you gained in this chapter that will help you name, define, and operationalize your concepts? Outline how you have connected the concepts in your project purpose statement to the concepts in your chosen framework.
> - *Essentials*: Review the advanced level competencies for the two *Essential* domains Systems-Based Practice and Knowledge for Nursing Practice. Reflect on how they relate to framing your clinical project.
> - *Project notebook addition*: Include a one-page written reflection that addresses your project purpose and chosen project concepts. Include the conceptual map or framework you are using to guide your project and the rationale for its use.

## SUMMARY AND KEY POINTS

Conscious use of appropriate concepts and theories/conceptual models will strengthen your own project as well as the body of scholarly work in nursing. The theoretical aspects of your project provide an overall framework that informs all three elements—purpose, methods, outcomes—of the project triangle. For example, the theory/conceptual model chosen (including its conceptual definitions) must match the way in which evaluation instruments used to collect data in your project define the concepts. Choosing the best framework for your project will help provide important guidance as the project moves forward. Points to recall from this chapter include the following:

- Concepts, theories, and conceptual models serve as frameworks to guide the clinical project and organize proposal writing.
- Theoretical and operational definitions provide project guidance and help clarify for all team members.
- These concepts, theories, and conceptual models (frameworks) establish the boundaries, structure and relationships, and concept definitions of your clinical project.
- Criteria for evaluating the appropriateness of potential frameworks include scope, context, logic, assumptions, usefulness, and simplicity.
- There are numerous nursing and nonnursing theories that can serve as project frameworks.

## WEBSITES FOR FURTHER REVIEW

Several websites that house repositories of project titles and abstracts are mentioned in the chapter. Additional examples of projects may be found online:

- *Virginia Henderson Global Nursing e-Repository*:
  https://library.mskcc.org/blog/2018/11/virginia-henderson-global-nursing-e-repository/
- *Sigma Repository*:
  www.sigmarepository.org

## NEXT CHAPTER UP

Now that you have identified the purpose of your project and have framed it within a theory/conceptual model, you are ready to identify the outcomes for your clinical project. Outcomes are one of the three key elements of the project triangle and are extremely important as they provide the focus for your entire clinical project. The outcomes need to be based on the clinical problem you want to address and will provide the foundation for the project's purpose statement and methods.

> **ONLINE/CLASSROOM DISCUSSION**
>
> In discussion with your classmates, share responses to the following questions:
>
> - What ways might you use the systems model of structure, process, and outcomes framework to begin outlining your project plans? What if there is interest in developing a diabetes clinic in a rural setting? How could this systems approach (or another framework) help you outline tentative project needs? What other theories/conceptual models might also be used to guide these projects?

## LEARNING ACTIVITIES

### To-Do List

1. Consider your planned project purpose and identify three concepts that are important to consider.
2. Scan the literature and your past textbooks. Identify and list at least three potential theories/conceptual frameworks that could relate to your project's purpose statement.
3. Consider how each of the preceding has potential value in your project. Pay particular attention to the concepts and how they are defined. What direction does this framework provide you?
4. Identify your choices to guide your project and justify your decision.

### Reflective Prompts

Questions to guide your thinking about how to frame your project include the following:

1. What conceptual model/framework are you planning to use in your project?
2. Why is the framework appropriate for this project?
3. Does the framework fit the scope and purpose of the project?
4. Does the framework provide useful guidance regarding the scope of the project?
5. Are all of the key elements of the purpose statement represented in the framework?
6. Is the framework simple in nature and easy to understand?
7. How will the clinical project benefit from using the framework?

### Activity

Using guidelines from the *National Strategy for Quality Improvement in Health Care* (U.S. Centers for Medicare & Medicaid Services, 2011), which concepts, models, or theories can you think of that could help you further your review of the literature or plan for an evidence-based project related to the following areas? Brainstorm with colleagues the pros and cons of the select concepts, conceptual models, or theories for each listed item.

- Make care safer by reducing the harm that results from faulty care systems.
- Ensure that each person and family is engaged as a partner in care.
- Promote effective communication and coordination of care.
- Promote the most effective prevention and treatment practices for the leading causes of mortality, starting with cardiovascular disease.
- Work with communities to promote wide use of best practices to enable healthy living.
- Make quality care more affordable for individuals, families, employers, and governments by developing and spreading new healthcare delivery models.

_____

_____

_____

_____

_____

_____

_____

_____

## REFERENCES

Chinn, P. L., & Kramer, M. K. (2019). *Knowledge development in nursing: Theory and process* (10th ed.). Elsevier Mosby.

McEwen, M., & Wills, W. M. (2019). *Theoretical basis for nursing* (5th ed.). Wolters Kluwer/Lippincott Williams & Wilkins.

Meleis, A. I. (2018). *Theoretical nursing: Development & progress* (6th ed.). Wolters Kluwer/Lippincott Williams & Wilkins.

Morton, A. (2012). What nurses need to know about sleep apnea. *Nursing Made Incredibly Easy*, *10*(3), 34–42. https://nursing.ceconnection.com/ovidfiles/00152258-201205000-00008.pdf

New York State Department of Health. (2020). *The model for improvement: Five critical components*. https://www.health.ny.gov/statistics/chac/improvement/components.htm

Peterson, S. J., & Bredow, T. S. (2020). *Middle range theories: Application to nursing research* (5th ed.). Wolters Kluwer/Lippincott Williams & Wilkins.

Rice, J., & Haycraft, K. (2012). Applying Lean and Six Sigma to your dermatology practice. *Journal of the Dermatology Nurses' Association*, *4*(2), 136–142. https://doi.org/10.1097/JDN.0b013e31824ab91e

U.S. Centers for Medicare & Medicaid Services. (2011). *Report to Congress: National strategy for quality improvement in health care*. https://www.cms.gov/cciio/resources/forms-reports-and-other-resources/quality03212011a

Walker, L., & Avant, K. (2019). *Strategies for theory construction in nursing* (6th ed.). Prentice Hall.

# SECTION II

## Writing Your Proposal: Designing and Setting the Stage for Your Project

# 8. Addressing Outcomes Evaluation in the Advanced Clinical Project Proposal

## INITIAL THOUGHT

"Outcomes: Which? When? Why? And how?"

## CHAPTER CONTENT

- Reflective Questions
- Quality Improvement Alert
- Considering Project Outcomes and Evaluation
- Outcomes and Concept Definitions
- Outcomes and Purpose (Aims) Statements
- Systems Models and Outcomes
  - Describing Your Outcomes Context
  - Backward Design
- Outcomes Evaluation and the Project Triangle
- Project Planning for Outcomes Evaluation
  - Naming Clear and Useful Outcomes Prospectively
  - Determining if Outcomes Are Reasonably Accessible
  - Identifying Timelines for When to Evaluate
  - Addressing the "So What" Factor for Outcomes
- Other Outcome Evaluation Considerations
- Technology and Outcomes Data
- Clinical Unit Policy Updates as Outcome Considerations
- Broad Outcome Evaluation Principles
- Tips for Getting Started
- Practice Scholarship Applications
- Summary and Key Points
- Websites for Further Review
- Next Chapter Up
- Online/Classroom Discussion
- Learning Activities
  - Outcomes and Your Experiences

## REFLECTIVE QUESTIONS

In Chapter 7, you learned about reviewing and considering theories or frameworks as a component of your clinical project and making them consistent with your project purpose. This chapter addresses outcome choices. Outcomes are one of the three key elements of the project triangle. The following reflective questions organize learning for this chapter. With which of the following are you most confident?

- Can you identify approaches to gaining project outcomes?
- What are the benefits/challenges to seeking selected project outcomes?
- Are you ready to begin a practical plan for project outcomes?

Use the Practice Scholarship Applications (at the end of this chapter) to help document your learning from concept to competency, including the relevant American Association of Colleges of Nursing (AACN) *Essentials* (2021).

This chapter focuses on an overview of project outcomes and basic principles of evaluating outcomes. For a good project, the concepts of interest should be clearly named and described, and reasonable evaluation approaches described. There are additional practical considerations; for instance, what will others do with the information and how likely will they be to use this information? This chapter addresses common outcomes considerations, the "outcomes" point on the project triangle, and outcomes as part of a systems model.

## QUALITY IMPROVEMENT ALERT

Outcomes for a QI project can be similar to other types of project outcomes. The focus for QI outcomes is typically relevant to a systems model that describes the structure and processes that lead to select outcomes.

## CONSIDERING PROJECT OUTCOMES AND EVALUATION

To evaluate outcomes means to determine how well a project achieved its objectives. Challenges can exist in naming outcomes and making evaluation plans. Some outcomes will be easier to name than others and even then, a variety of approaches for operationalizing these exist. For example, even ways to evaluate patient educational outcomes such as knowledge and application are very different (a true/false quiz might evaluate knowledge gain, but an application of knowledge would include something more consistent with patient observation or application to a case). Evaluating outcomes, naming the outcomes to be evaluated and how these would be appraised, are key components of quality improvement (QI) models.

## OUTCOMES AND CONCEPT DEFINITIONS

You will want to be very specific about the outcomes chosen and how they will be evaluated or measured. This includes clearly naming each outcome and then determining how best to define and evaluate that outcome. As discussed in Chapter 7, this is similar to concept analysis and relates to naming, defining, and operationalizing a specific concept. The terms "theoretical" (naming and defining) and "operational" (how the concept will be evaluated) definitions are used. This needs to be done prospectively so that you establish clearly how the outcomes will be evaluated. Often these concepts and definitions are addressed as components of a conceptual framework or project conceptual map. In general:

- You will want to identify outcomes that are as concrete as is reasonable for your concept. Some concepts are easier to gain true measures of than others. For example, physiological measures, such as blood glucose, are typically recognized as having good reliability and validity. Other measures, such as self-reported dietary intake, are typically considered less reliable. There are differences in how objectively different outcomes are measured.

- In another example, physical exercise tolerance measures are more concrete than self-reported exercise behaviors on a patient self-survey. That does not mean there is no value to each measure, but in the proposal, you will make choices and need to defend why you chose select approaches to evaluate outcomes.

You will be as specific as possible in your choices of outcomes evaluation, noting, for example, whether you will evaluate self-reported weight change versus weight change on clinical exam scale records. Additionally, note that there can be challenges with *ambiguous terms*. If your project involves concepts such as "increased access" for "high-risk" patients, you will need to be very clear on what these terms mean. What is the general consensus for defining the outcome of increased access? Do high risk patients mean those with elevation of selected labs? What does each term mean specifically for this project? Other outcomes, such as knowledge, satisfaction, and behaviors, will present their own definition challenges. Clarity and consistency in using these terms in your proposal are needed.

## OUTCOMES AND PURPOSE (AIMS) STATEMENTS

As will be discussed in Chapter 9, purpose statements or aims guide the project including the project outcomes choices. Clinical projects typically consider outcomes of interest, rather than dependent variables found in research. While a research hypothesis identifies expected study outcomes as the dependent variable (i.e., what is being measured or observed), in clinical projects, the project purpose statement (or aims statement) is used to name expected project outcomes.

All named outcomes should relate to your purpose statement, but how you evaluate these outcomes can vary. Your population focus can suggest the need for diverse outcomes. For example, if you are interested in health promotion outcomes it makes sense to consider your specific populations and targeted outcomes.

- Health promotion outcomes for an adolescent population are likely quite different than for older adults, so focus on those that are important to your specific population.

- Targeted outcomes also vary by targets and set criteria. For example, you may not want "all or nothing" targets for outcomes. For example, if patients are frail older adults with diabetes and congestive heart failure, what does "health promotion" mean for them? What is the specific target for health promotion? Can it be defined in terms of patient function? How broad or how specific will this be?

- In some cases, you will be considering comparisons to outcomes criteria set by external agencies such as Healthy People 2030. For example, how do patients with diabetes in your population compare to national population guides? Thinking ahead about important outcomes helps focus project purpose and methods (the additional project triangle points).

## SYSTEMS MODELS AND OUTCOMES

Systems frameworks are well respected in QI and other evidence-based projects. Systems provide direction in describing context for your outcomes, even in considering a project from a backwards design perspective.

### Describing Your Outcomes Context

A systems model can help describe the context for your project outcomes. For example, as healthcare providers, you are working in very complex healthcare settings. A systems model, focusing on structure/process/outcomes, is very helpful in naming, managing, and evaluating the multiple components of such complex settings. Part of outcomes evaluation is first naming your *outcome* of interest and then describing the *structure* (resources) and the *process* (activities) or what you do to seek these outcomes. This means considering outcomes as part of a systems framework. Naming outcomes in isolation, without considering the context of structure and process, prevents others from seeing the full picture (Health Resources and Services Administration [HRSA], n.d.).

## Backward Design

Backward design can be used in considering your systems approach. It provides the opportunity to first identify the outcomes that you are seeking and then working backward to name the needed structure and process for project design. For example, if your project includes seeking improved staff knowledge about a topic, knowing the specific outcomes you are going for helps you focus on the structure and process needed for the educational project. (Seeking the right program structure and process can help address what some of the issues may be for the program's successes or failures.)

## OUTCOMES EVALUATION AND THE PROJECT TRIANGLE

Outcomes are a major focus with a clinical project and the project triangle (Appendix A) is key in helping to align the many project components. Part of this process is making outcome choices fit with data collection methods. In the project triangle, the purpose statement, methods, and outcomes represent the three points that need to mesh; a key feature of evaluation and outcomes is keeping these three components (purpose, methods, and outcomes) aligned with one another.

In a broad example, a staff education department wants to demonstrate that their programs impact staff knowledge and behaviors (*purpose*). They begin by developing and implementing an evidence-based educational session (*methods*) and then evaluate staff knowledge gain and behavior change with specific measures (*outcomes*).

As you revisit the project triangle, start by keeping concepts broad and simple, then work toward the level of detail needed for the desired project. Similar to concept analysis, name the outcomes you are going for, define them, and then operationalize them.

## PROJECT PLANNING FOR OUTCOMES EVALUATION

When considering outcomes evaluation, basic concepts can be useful in making project planning choices. Some points to consider include those described in the following paragraphs.

### Naming Clear and Useful Outcomes Prospectively

Clear and useful outcomes provide focus and benefit. As you cannot ask and answer all evaluative questions, the challenge is to choose useful outcomes data. These data can guide you in gaining the correct data rather than a lot of extraneous data. Avoid collecting data for their own sake. You do not want to spend time collecting large amounts of evaluation data that will just be stored in an electronic filing cabinet. So this involves thinking ahead about who the users are, whether the data address issues that are important to the users, and whether the data can be presented in a clear understandable format for the users.

### Determining if Outcomes Are Reasonably Accessible

Consideration should include whether the outcomes will be reasonably accessible. What practical data already exist? Can you gain ideas for outcomes measures from data sources or reports that are already in place? Data sets are often available that could have relevance to your project, often found in completed needs assessments or formal reports generated for accreditation or other purposes. Reviewing similar resources in your settings and determining what is easily available can be helpful steps in your planning. Key tips to address if you will be working within a specific unit/organization include the following:

- Collaborate with the organization to determine what data will be useful to them.
- Set up meetings with key personnel to determine what measures matter to them. They can provide clarity to the focus of data collection and analysis for your project. Make sure you can access data and if those data can be shared.
- Determine what resources you will have access to including what data can be collected, who will collect the data, and how the data will be collected.
- Consider proprietary information and have a conversation about what information and data can be shared outside the organization. For instance, some organizations will only allow aggregate data to be shared and the organization must be de-identified.
- Work with your mentor to determine if data will be reasonably available to evaluate selected outcomes.

### Identifying Timelines for When to Evaluate

You should also consider relevant time factors for your planned outcomes. Outcomes evaluation, described as addressing impacts of a program or intervention, can be considered from short-, medium-, and long-term perspectives (HRSA, n.d.). Clinical projects typically first address short-term outcomes and then use a follow-up plan to address long-term outcomes. You will also determine whether baseline data exist or need to be collected. The proposal needs to document these decisions specifically. How much time will you have to collect data? Can selected outcomes be easily measured in the time frame? For example, after nutrition education teaching, you cannot measure a reduction in cardiovascular risk over 3 months, but you can measure a reduction in weight or triglycerides.

- Clarify benchmarks versus target outcomes. A baseline value is your current performance level. Now you want to aim for your desired performance. Benchmarks are a comparison point against external standards. Targets provide the specific outcomes that you plan to achieve within a certain timeframe.
- Are you seeking to meet a set benchmark such as an increase or decrease in your outcome value? If so, do you have data that have been collected prior to your project to compare to?
- Or are you trying to achieve a target with a new intervention (e.g., you want to achieve a 75% completion rate on a screening tool that is new to the clinic)?

### Addressing the "So What" Factor for Outcomes

Many factors inform the outcomes that are identified for any given clinical project. These include, among other things, the purpose of your project, the methods of your project (both of which are illustrated by the triangle), and outcomes of particular interest. They can relate to patient outcomes, staff outcomes, or systems outcomes. As you consider potential outcomes, the "so what" question is important and can be further clarified by addressing questions such as the following:

- What will others do with the outcomes?
- What difference will the project make in improving health, education, or healthcare quality, costs, and, most important, patient, family, or community outcomes?
- Is there a probability that this project outcome is relevant to others from a feasibility and reproducibility perspective?

## OTHER OUTCOME EVALUATION CONSIDERATIONS

Broad unit or population outcomes are important considerations. Making a case for stakeholders and showing unit accountability as a whole relates to the value of a clinical project. For example, in staff development the purpose is typically to document staff competency and gain good agency outcomes. Systems models, as previously noted, allow you to document the structure and process used for gaining these.

- As one student noted for a rehabilitation unit project:
  *Our nursing staff is concerned about positive outcomes for our patient populations who have strokes. Using a systems model we described the unit structure and process. Using an evidence-based assessment tool to monitor patient outcomes, we use the National Institute of Health Stroke Scale as a type of premeasure when a patient is first hospitalized after an acute stroke, and then again at discharge from the hospital to monitor functional levels. Also, as part of this system, all nursing staff have to demonstrate competency in using the stroke assessment tool at least yearly. We can show outcomes and staff support for this ongoing project.*
- Related to clinical unit and financial outcomes, your proposal should also make a case for stakeholders, showing that you are considering costs and efficiency to demonstrate accountability. Common measures include cost savings, cost avoidance, and revenue generation.

## TECHNOLOGY AND OUTCOMES DATA

Diverse opportunities for gaining outcome data exist. Technology with large data sets as well as common electronic tools used in scholarly projects are examples.

Often you can use some type of electronic data collection tools for surveys, interviews, observations, or document reviews. Versions of these tools include both qualitative and quantitative approaches to gaining data. These varied data collection methods will need to be described in your proposal as such, with strengths and limits of each noted. Chapters 11 and 12 address these strategies, including how you will name the tools for measuring your concepts or outcomes of interest. Although variations exist in each of these approaches, these options provide a good starting point for considering the ideal and real possibilities for evaluating project outcomes.

Technology and large data sets are good considerations when making outcomes choices. In some cases, technology can make data collection easier; for example:

- Document reviews include accessing data from electronic records, equivalent to patient charts, or electronic clinical log documentation such as Typhon. Reviewing these data for themes can lead to needed project support (or later to help with analyses).
- Technology often fits with large available data sets. In the long-term care setting, for example, the minimum data set (MDS) for accessing resident outcomes includes the opportunity to evaluate your sample's outcomes against recommended standards. These data can also be grouped with other patient records and can then be compared, not only by individual patient records, but also with facilities at state and national levels. The MDS outcomes (such as weight loss), are captured first on individual patients as part of their electronic record, and then evaluated against an evidence-based national standard.
- Additionally similar opportunities exist with acute care databases such as the Agency for Healthcare Research and Quality (AHRQ) Quality Indicators and Hospital Inpatient Quality Measures. Tools such as these can be used by hospitals to identify potential problem areas needing further study. Additionally they can be used to help assess quality of care (www.ahrq.gov/sites/default/files/wysiwyg/professionals/systems/hospital/qitoolkit/combined/a1a_combo_iqifactsheet.pdf).

## CLINICAL UNIT POLICY UPDATES AS OUTCOME CONSIDERATIONS

Why consider clinical policy change as a potential project outcome? These clinical policies or sets of recommendations for the care of patients with specific conditions can lead to guidance for safe, quality care. Consider the following as potential approaches to develop new or enhance current clinical policies as outcomes.

- Will your project help identify important clinical issues/processes that could potentially lead to improvement with a current policy revision or a new policy?
- Could evidence-based changes to a current policy improve patient care and (further health outcomes) or lead to policy development that guides safe, effective, and efficient care?
- Beyond your clinical agency, would sharing your project provide for potential policy resources for similar clinical units or even allow input for broader healthcare policies?

## BROAD OUTCOME EVALUATION PRINCIPLES

Evaluation principles are important considerations in your outcome choices. As you begin to make plans to evaluate chosen outcomes, a list of principles that can guide outcome evaluation plans is described by the American Association of Higher Education (AAHE, n.d.). Although these have been framed from a student-evaluation perspective, the principles apply to staff development, and, in most cases, patient care evaluation as well. These have been determined to be a form of best evaluation practices. Of note, there is value in multiple-method approaches that provide a type of triangulation to evaluation. Using varied methods, as well as gaining differing perspectives from those in varied positions, can add to the credibility of outcomes data evaluation plans. The principles described by the AAHE (n.d.) are paraphrased in the following list. They note that outcome evaluation works best when the following conditions are met:

- It begins with broad values statements, or core principles which in essence describe the purpose of the evaluation.
- It comes from integrated, multiple perspectives and is considered over time.
- Purposes are clearly stated.
- It addresses not only the outcomes, but also the processes that lead to these.
- It is ongoing (as in QI) rather than episodic.
- Multiple team members are involved.
- It involves practical issues that are important to people.
- It is used for improvements as part of a larger set of change initiatives.
- It meets responsibilities to the public as well as agency stakeholders.

## TIPS FOR GETTING STARTED

As you proceed with your clinical project, here are some questions to ask:

- What outcomes would you and your clinical organization like your clinical project to achieve? How can these outcomes impact your clinical setting or patient population?
- Will your outcomes be relevant? For example, if you are working within a specific unit, ask if the measure tells the organization what it needs to know. The measure needs to matter, informing and providing evidence of success or needed change.
- What evaluation data are you already gaining in your clinical setting? Which are most helpful in documenting outcomes? Gaining current, baseline data to see where these outcomes stand provides a good starting point for evaluation.
- Will these outcomes be short term? Long term? What challenges still exist? Will you have time to evaluate? What is still needed? Are these outcomes reasonable and realistic? Concrete and attainable?

### PRACTICE SCHOLARSHIP APPLICATIONS

Consider your competency documentation plans. How will your project address select *Essentials*? Consider additions to your project notebook as you complete the following:

- *Concepts to competence*: In reviewing Chapters 7 and 8, how will you operationalize your concepts of interest? Review the Reflective Questions from the beginning of the chapter and self-assess on your progress with this chapter as you begin your work.
- *Essentials*: Review advanced level competencies and subcompetencies for the *Essentials* domains Systems-Based Practice, Knowledge for Nursing Practice, Quality and Safety, and Population Health, and reflect on how they relate to your clinical project. How are these relevant to your planned DNP project and your professional career plans?
- *Project notebook*: Start with a one-page written reflection that addresses your project purpose and outcomes. Include potential outcomes choices and identify potential evaluation concerns. Using the project triangle, begin working backward from outcomes you are seeking to identify potential methods to evaluate.

## SUMMARY AND KEY POINTS

Naming clearly the desired practical project outcomes provides another step that moves the project forward. What is hoped for? What is to be gained? Outcomes evaluation is a key component of advanced clinical projects. Positive outcomes can show clinical accountability and serve as indicators of success. Projected outcomes are a point on the project triangle aligning with the project purpose and methods. Points to recall from this chapter include the following:

- It is important to consider outcomes evaluation as you begin project planning.
- You will be identifying concept outcomes and defining them not only theoretically but also operationally.
- Outcomes vary by project purpose and targets (and outcomes vary by concepts of interest).
- Systems models can provide structure and context in relation to outcomes.
- Naming outcomes serves a purpose in clearly identifying project targets.
- Outcomes need to be identified prospectively; they should have specific timelines for indicating when to evaluate.
- Project considerations should include whether the outcomes will be reasonably accessible.
- Evaluation plans work best when based on broad outcome evaluation principles.
- Choices about outcomes should be a fit within your project triangle.

## WEBSITES FOR FURTHER REVIEW

Ideas for outcomes can be gained by reviewing resources at select websites such as national reports from the National Academy of Sciences. The following websites, for example, focus on health outcomes. Ideas for small-scale projects might be gained from these and similar national reports. For each of the following web resources reviewed, what surprises you? What might apply to your further work?

- Healthy People 2030, *Overall Health and Well-Being Measures*:

    https://health.gov/healthypeople/objectives-and-data/overall-health-and-well-being-measures

- *Toward Quality Measures for Population Health and the Leading Health Indicators*:

    https://nap.nationalacademies.org/catalog/18339/toward-quality-measures-for-population-health-and-the-leading-health-indicators

## NEXT CHAPTER UP

The next chapter focuses on naming a specific purpose statement for your plan. The purpose statement serves as a focus and type of contract for your project.

### ONLINE/CLASSROOM DISCUSSION

From a selection of potential project titles, which outcomes are clearest to you? What are the concepts? How would you consider theoretical and operational definitions for these concepts?

- early detection of heart failure
- diabetic control in the ICU
- falls in stroke patients
- outpatient management of diabetes mellitus

## LEARNING ACTIVITIES

### Outcomes and Your Experiences

Most nurses have participated in and are familiar with continuing education programs. Think of a recent program you attended and consider what outcomes were evaluated.

- Were the common approaches of knowledge gain, change in perspectives, or planned behavior change evident?
- Were there other outcomes that could have been gained to show value in the program?
- How would you name and describe those outcomes?
- What ways might you capture those outcomes: Knowledge test? Attitude survey? Planned behavior change survey? Satisfaction with the learning activity? Other?

## REFERENCES

American Association of Higher Education. (n.d.). *9 principles of good practice for assessing student learning.* https://www.dartmouth.edu/~oir/assessmenteval/tools/9principles.html

Health Resources and Services Administration. (n.d.). *Health workforce training program evaluation toolkit.* https://bhw.hrsa.gov/sites/default/files/bureau-health-workforce/funding/hrsa-pcte-toolkit-full.pdf

McNamara, C. (n.d.). *Basic guide to outcomes-based evaluation for nonprofit organizations with very limited resources.* https://managementhelp.org/evaluation/outcomes-evaluation-guide.htm

Whitman, G. (2003). What patient outcome should our outcomes management team measure? *Outcomes Management, 7*(3), 94–96.

# 9. Guiding the Advanced Clinical Project: The Purpose of a Purpose Statement

## INITIAL THOUGHT

"To be or not to be: What is the clinical project's reason for being?"

## CHAPTER CONTENT

- Reflective Questions
- Quality Improvement Alert
- What Is the Purpose Statement?
  - Semantics and the Purpose Statement
- The Project Triangle
- How Is a Purpose Statement Related to the Clinical Problem?
- Problem Statement to Purpose Statement
  - From Problem to Solution
  - Using the Clinical Question
  - Revising Your Purpose Statement and Putting It in Context
  - The Final Purpose Statement
- Checklist: Evaluating the Purpose Statement
- Peer Review of the Purpose Statement
- Advice From DNP Students
- Practice Scholarship Applications
- Summary and Key Points
- Websites for Further Review
- Next Chapter Up
- Online/Classroom Discussion
- Learning Activities
  - To-Do List

## REFLECTIVE QUESTIONS

In earlier chapters, you identified a clinical problem, and in Chapter 8 you identified an outcome that, if met, would resolve your clinical problem and improve care. In this chapter, you use your clinical problem and identified outcome to develop a purpose statement. The following reflective questions organize learning for this chapter. With which of the following are you most confident?

- What is a purpose statement?
- How are purpose statements, aims, objectives, and goals related?
- Why is a purpose statement important?
- How is a purpose statement related to the clinical problem, concepts, and outcomes?

Use the Practice Scholarship Applications (at the end of this chapter) to help document your learning from concept to competency, including the relevant American Association of Colleges of Nursing (AACN) *Essentials* (2021).

## QUALITY IMPROVEMENT ALERT

The purpose statement/aims provide direction and goals for the quality improvement (QI) project.

## WHAT IS THE PURPOSE STATEMENT?

In previous chapters, you identified potential outcomes for your clinical project. Now you will turn to writing the purpose statement, which will address the clinical problem and provide continued direction throughout the duration of the project. For example, if the clinical problem is inconsistency in orienting patients to cardiac rehabilitation, such that vital content is sometimes missed or care is not individualized enough, then the purpose statement should direct the project by addressing that problem and finding an answer. In this case, taking the problem statement to the next level includes generating a purpose statement that guides the project toward resolving the problem of cardiac rehabilitation orientation. You may have to consider solutions or strategies for further study of that problem, and these reflections will lead your thinking and writing to a clear purpose statement for your project. To illustrate, the purpose in the preceding example may be to develop a template to guide the development and testing of future new cardiac rehabilitation orientation exemplars.

### Semantics and the Purpose Statement

A good purpose statement flows from the problem statement and is a single sentence that states the general intent of the clinical project, including the context, so that it provides guidance and direction (Dusick, 2014). The project topic, population, methods, variables, and setting are incorporated.

Note that different organizations may use different terminology such as aims, goals, or objectives. There may be subtle distinctions among these terms according to specific organizations and funding agencies, or preferences for one name over another held by various graduate programs. For example, the National Institutes of Health do not refer to purpose statements, but rather to specific aims. Specific aims identify the goals and objectives of the proposed project by stating what will be done in the project, how it will be done, why it will be done, and the expected impact of the work (Principal Investigators Leader, 2018). Referred to as the purpose statement in this text, the SMART mnemonic (**S**pecific, **M**easurable, **A**chievable, **R**elevant, and **T**ime-bound) suggests approaches to incorporate in these guiding statements.

The fundamental reason for these statements is to build on answering a clinical question and providing direction for a problem solution. For the purposes of this book, the purpose statement and other noted terms are considered similar in their role of providing direction and guidance to the clinical project.

## THE PROJECT TRIANGLE

The purpose statement (again, also referred to as aims, goals, and objectives) provides guidance and direction throughout the project. The project triangle uses the purpose statement to ensure that the clinical problem is addressed and to keep all elements of the project consistent with one another and with the project as a whole. Recall that the three points of the triangle represent the purpose statement, methods, and outcomes. As you progress through the advanced clinical project, those three points should remain intact, indicating consistency among the purpose, methods, and outcomes. Note that the purpose statement is deliberately positioned at the top of the triangle; it might even be considered analogous to the North Star in providing direction and guidance throughout the project.

Your own proposal may be to develop evidence-based protocols for managing chronic health problems, to develop evidence-based education programs to guide staff in gaining competencies, or to generate new evidence related to unique patient population needs. Regardless of the project proposed, there will undoubtedly be times of confusion and misdirection as you progress. At these times, remember the project triangle and purpose statement, as they are essential in redirecting focus back to the proposed project.

For example, lost in the volumes of literature on cardiac rehabilitation, you may find yourself reviewing evidence relating to pediatrics and wondering whether that is how you should be spending your time. Return to the purpose statement and determine whether the population identified includes pediatrics or not. If adults are specified in the purpose statement, then you need to redirect your literature review to focus on adults. When you lose direction or begin to flounder, look to the top of the triangle and review the purpose statement. The rest of the project should be consistent with and support that purpose statement.

## HOW IS A PURPOSE STATEMENT RELATED TO THE CLINICAL PROBLEM?

You identified an outcome in Chapter 8 that, if achieved, would address your clinical problem and improve the quality of patient care. The next step is to take that clinical problem statement and outcome and translate them into a purpose statement. In the purpose statement you take an existing clinical problem statement and translate it into a statement that will guide you into a future resolution (outcome) of the problem. Thus, addressing the purpose statement will answer the clinical problem identified (Dusick, 2014) and produce the desired outcome.

Just as naming the problem and reviewing the literature occurs together, as discussed in earlier chapters, the development of the purpose statement also occurs simultaneously with the literature review. As the purpose statement represents the future answer to a current clinical problem, it is important that current information about the problem is known and accounted for in the project. It is also important that enough literature be reviewed to establish the clinical relevance and value of the proposed clinical project. When completed and reviewed, the purpose statement should confirm the focus and value of the clinical project in terms of addressing the identified problem statement and also contributing to the best current evidence in clinical practice.

## PROBLEM STATEMENT TO PURPOSE STATEMENT

### From Problem to Solution

You are now ready to move from a clinical problem that needs to be addressed to improve patient care (your problem statement) to a project purpose that will help solve that problem (your purpose statement). For example, the lack of evidence supporting the use of simulation in the hospital orientation of new graduates may be the problem to solve, and generating evidence about the effectiveness of simulation experiences to guide graduate nurses in the 3-month, new hospital employee orientation would be an appropriate way to state the purpose that would address that problem.

Although it is preferable for purpose statements to provide details of the project, it may be helpful to first practice the transition from problem statement to general-purpose statement, than from problem to solution. Recall the nurse who did not have a consistent or thorough orientation for new cardiac rehabilitation patients. Think about what the solution to that problem would be in order to start writing the purpose statement. In this case, the purpose statement might be to conduct a comprehensive literature review in order to establish a new orientation protocol (and implement that protocol and evaluate). Do you see the transition from a clinical problem (an inconsistent orientation for new cardiac rehabilitation patients) to a project that addresses the problem (a literature review to establish an orientation protocol)? Another example might be as follows: You are using simulation to orient new graduate nurses to the hospital, but you are not sure whether you are using an effective method of orientation. That problem might translate into the following project purpose statement: The purpose of this project is to generate evidence regarding the effectiveness of the simulation experiences for new nursing staff and to identify implications for future orientation sessions.

## Using the Clinical Question

When moving from the clinical problem to the purpose statement, you are moving from a problem that needs to be solved to a future project that will address that problem. Sometimes a helpful step in moving from the clinical problem statement to the purpose statement is to first convert the clinical problem into a clinical question, which implies a future response and, in turn, represents your project's purpose. In addition to helping you clarify the desired outcomes of your advanced clinical project, the clinical question can also provide a reasonable starting point for a literature search. Note that the way the clinical problem is stated makes a big difference in the topic that is addressed and the answer that will be found.

For example, Melnyk and Fineout-Overholt's (2023) **P**opulation, **I**ntervention, **C**omparison, **O**utcome, and **T**ime (PICOT) questions provide a sample format that demonstrates this principle for reviewing the literature. Perhaps you have implemented simulations into the hospital orientation for new nurses, and the clinical problem you need to address is whether use of simulations provides an adequate orientation experience. Note the nuances in the following questions and the answers that will be produced.

- For graduate nurses taking a 3-month, new hospital employee orientation program, how do clinical experiences versus simulated experiences affect skill acquisition and critical thinking skills?
- For graduate nurses taking a 3-month, new hospital employee orientation program, do simulated experiences compared with clinical experiences lead to more accuracy identifying at-risk, new graduate employees?
- How do graduate nurses in a 3-month, new hospital employee orientation program perceive or value simulated experiences?

The PICO question serves well in many situations, such as those concerned with best treatments for patients, healthcare interventions, and experimental research. However, it may not fit other topics (such as systems of care, program effectiveness, policies, QI, and management issues) quite as well. While there are a number of different formats used to ask clinical questions, another general format for clinical questions is the **P**roblem, **P**opulation, **C**hange, **O**utcome (PPCO) question (Waldrop & Jennings-Dunlap, 2024). PPCO questions emphasize both the background of the problem in general as well as in the local context. Next the population affected by the problem is stated and then the change element that research has shown to help address the problem is identified. Finally, the outcome (i.e., the observable difference made by the change) is stated. A sample PPCO question is: When dehydration prompts presentation to the emergency department (P) in the frail elderly (P), what measures can be taken (C) to reduce readmission (O)?

Again, PICOT and PPCO questions may guide your literature search and help you identify the level of literature/research evidence available relevant to the clinical problem you have identified. In fact, they may be most useful in guiding the literature review, rather than providing further project direction, because of the limited number of well-developed studies in so many diverse areas of nursing. Now reflect on the three clinical questions just posed in this section and consider the purpose statement that might flow from each. For example, if your clinical question is about how graduate nurses perceive simulated experiences, then your purpose statements for each format would be different (as follows):

- *PICO*: The purpose of this project is to describe how graduate nurses perceive simulated experiences as part of their 3-month, new hospital employee orientation program.
- *PPCO*: When participating in simulated experiences as part of a 3-month, new hospital employee orientation program for graduate nurses, what actions can be taken to achieve positive perceptions of the simulation experience?

Remember that different clinical problems and questions can lead to various purpose statements and outcomes; therefore, make sure you write the purpose statement that answers the question you really want to have answered.

## Revising Your Purpose Statement and Putting It in Context

Keep in mind that the first draft of your purpose statement will not be your final purpose statement. The initial leap from problem statement to general purpose statement is a vital exercise in transitioning from the current problem to the future project solution. However, once that initial step is taken, there will likely be multiple iterations as you move from an initial purpose statement to a fully mature and well-expressed purpose statement.

Also, be aware that revising your initial statement into a good purpose statement is harder than it might seem at first glance. Take, for example, the following statement: The purpose of this project is to develop a teaching tool for new hospital nurses. This statement leaves the reader with more questions than answers: What is the topic of the teaching tool? A teaching tool for a skills lab would be very different from a teaching tool about hospital policies. What level of new nurses? A teaching tool for new graduates would be very different from one for seasoned nurses. Once you have an initial purpose statement written, read it over several times and ask yourself what is missing. That missing information provides direction for your subsequent purpose statement revisions. After considering the following purpose statements, identify *missing* information, and revise each statement to provide the missing information. The purpose of this clinical project is to

- implement a new simulation scenario for clinical nurses,
- improve the quality of care for patients hospitalized in the Midwest, and
- evaluate peer-led support groups for newly diagnosed teenage diabetics.

The need for repeated revisions of the purpose statement is quite common. In each of the preceding statements, can you identify the topic, concepts, methods, population, setting, and the outcomes? In the first statement, for example, the topic is simulation, and that is the only concept that is identified. The method is not mentioned. The population is clinical nurses, but which clinical nurses and the setting are not identified. The outcome is a new simulation scenario. Without more information about the concepts, methods, population and setting, it is difficult to understand what will be done in this project and why. A more complete purpose statement provides much more detail and direction: The purpose of this clinical project is to develop and implement an evidence-based simulation scenario with rubric, focusing on the clinical use of a new bed safety product to measure ICU staff nurses' application in patient care. Now, consider the remaining two purposes statements presented earlier and, determine what content is missing, and write (and rewrite) revised purposes statements.

## The Final Purpose Statement

Although it would be nice for purpose statements to answer every who, what, when, where, and how question, sometimes that is not feasible. Minimally, the purpose statement should be honed down to a single concise statement, written explicitly as the purpose statement, which identifies the project topic and population. Preferably it will also include the methods to be used, variables involved, and the setting (Cambridge Rindge & Latin School, 2009; Dusick, 2014). An example of a good purpose statement is as follows: The purpose of this project is to develop an evidence-based protocol regarding the use of simulation experiences to optimize skill acquisition in a 3-month, new graduate nurse hospital-orientation program. Note that this purpose statement includes the topic (simulation), method (evidence gathered from a review of literature), the concepts (simulation and skill acquisition), the population (new graduate nurses), the setting (hospital orientation), and the outcome (skill acquisition). Again, reflect on the nuances of this purpose statement and the way in which subtle changes might affect the nature of the project and the outcomes obtained.

The final question to ask yourself as you revise and refine your purpose statement is this: If I conduct this project, will the clinical problem I started with be addressed or resolved? Assuming skill acquisition and critical thinking are the two outcomes you are interested in, this purpose statement will produce an outcome that answers the clinical problem originally identified so you are ready to move forward to map out your clinical project. But if not, stop now before investing more time in the wrong project and back up to your clinical problem. Rework the previous steps, explore the fine nuances in the clinical question you want to answer, and rewrite the purpose statement until it describes the work you need to do to resolve the clinical problem you initially identified.

## CHECKLIST: EVALUATING THE PURPOSE STATEMENT

Recall that the problem statement and outcome are inextricably linked to the purpose statement. After you have written an initial purpose statement, revised it, and decided on your final version, then answer the following yes-or-no questions:

1. Are you attempting to solve the right problem? Have you looked at the issue from multiple perspectives (such as people, place, and process factors) and considered the best approach for focusing your project?
2. Is the project purpose stated completely? Does it incorporate the proposed population, any proposed intervention, and proposed outcomes?
3. Have you read enough literature relevant to your topic to know that your project purpose has relevance?
4. Is it clear how the project will be limited or focused to make it manageable?

5. Does the purpose statement have the potential to provide important and useful information to improve clinical practice?
6. Will the purpose statement lead to the desired outcome?
7. Is the purpose focused enough to be accomplished with a reasonable expenditure of time, money, and effort?
8. Have you considered potential pitfalls?
9. Will the project have the potential to advance clinical processes or outcomes in an important way?
10. Is this project really what you want to focus on?

If you answer each question with a resounding yes, then you are ready to move forward. Any no responses indicate a need for further reflection and likely additional revisions to the purpose statement.

## PEER REVIEW OF THE PURPOSE STATEMENT

There are two additional steps in writing a good purpose statement. First, continue to review your purpose statement and make appropriate revisions and repeat this activity on several different occasions. Time does make a difference, so when you believe you have your final purpose statement, come back to it at several different times to make sure it still passes the yes/no questions checklist.

Second, ask a colleague to review your purpose statement and provide feedback. Give this step serious thought, considering the strengths various colleagues have to offer in this process, and decide on those who have the most to offer. Choose peers who will provide honest, if gentle, constructive criticism rather than those who will just provide the easier-to-give (and receive) compliments. With an initial list in hand, begin a thorough process of identifying the best candidates to recruit for this important job:

- What are the person's strengths in terms of content?
- What are the person's strengths in terms of interpersonal skills?
- What limitations does the person have in terms of time, content, and interactions?
- Will the person provide honest feedback?
- Are there other factors to consider?

An objective peer review will likely result in needed revisions that you would otherwise miss. Have more than one person review the purpose statement, preferably a nurse and a nonnurse colleague both, as this will provide a broader review and greater variety of perspectives. Keep in mind that this step may take more time than expected, depending on your reviewers' respective schedules, so build that time into your own project timeline. Also keep in mind the thoughts of previous DNP students as they wrestled with their own purpose statements, as presented in Advice From DNP Students box.

### ADVICE FROM DNP STUDENTS

**Purpose Statements**

Use the purpose statement to keep your project focused.

- The most important thing I learned was how to narrow the focus of my project.

Keep the purpose statement in front of you at all times.

- Keep the purpose of the project in mind.
- If the beginning section of the project is not aligned (correctly focused with the purpose), then the entire project is misaligned.
- From general idea to specific problem, writing a succinct purpose statement—including the concepts in a context—becomes clear as the proposal unfolds.

### PRACTICE SCHOLARSHIP APPLICATIONS

Consider your competency documentation plans. How will your project address select *Essentials*? Consider additions to your project notebook as you complete the following.

- *Concepts to competence*: Think about your knowledge of purpose statements. Describe the critical thinking process by which you moved from your clinical problem statement to the purpose statement, as well as how the completed purpose statement is consistent with the project methods and outcomes (as presented in the project triangle).
- *Essentials*: Review the advanced-level domain competencies of the Knowledge for Nursing Practice and Scholarship for the Nursing Discipline *Essential* domains. Reflect on how they relate to writing a good purpose statement.
- *Project notebook*: Complete a one-sentence purpose statement that clearly communicates the intent of your project. Include a reflection on your perception of the strengths and weaknesses of this statement.

## SUMMARY AND KEY POINTS

This chapter has provided a thorough guide in moving your problem statement to the purpose statement you will use for your proposal. Consider the significance of the purpose statement and its importance to clinical practice. Would you be enthused about working on this proposal? If it were addressed, would patient care be improved? Points to recall from this chapter include the following:

- Purpose statements go by many names—aims, goals, and objectives—and in this book the purpose statement is considered similar to those terms.
- The purpose statement provides direction throughout the project and is essential to maintaining the integrity of the project triangle that supports the project.
- Clinical questions can be useful tools in transitioning from a problem statement to a purpose statement. The purpose statement takes an existing clinical problem statement and translates it into a statement that will lead to future resolution of that problem.
- Be prepared to revise your purpose statement multiple times.
- Review the final purpose statement to be sure it includes the project topic, population, methods, variables, and setting.

## WEBSITES FOR FURTHER REVIEW

How others have focused purpose statements and project questions can be helpful in gaining ideas and thinking through your own project. Examples of resources used to gain further ideas about purpose statements and project questions can be found at the following websites:

- East Carolina University Libraries, *Asking the Clinical Question*:

  https://libguides.ecu.edu/c.php?g=17486&p=97639
- University of Missouri, *Using PICO Questions*:

  https://libraryguides.missouri.edu/c.php?g=28271&p=174073

## NEXT CHAPTER UP

You now have a clearly written purpose statement that links your project to a clinical problem and guides your project as it resolves that problem by attaining the desired outcome. The next step is to map out your clinical project, from the purpose statement to the findings, including all of the intervening activities. Remember that the methods and data-collection plans must remain consistent with the problem, outcomes, and purpose statement. Also keep in mind that, although anticipating potential problems and laying the groundwork for your final project paper takes more time now, both will prove to be the most efficient means of implementing and completing your clinical project.

## LEARNING ACTIVITIES

### To-Do List

1. Think back to Chapter 3 when you identified potential clinical problems and wrote problem statements. Select three of your ideas from that chapter and take the leap from the problem statement (which you previously wrote) to an initial purpose statement. Evaluate your initial purpose statement by asking yourself the following two questions:
   - Do you see the transition from an existing clinical problem to a project that, if conducted, would address that clinical problem?
   - If the project were conducted, would it solve your clinical problem?
2. Go back to your three initial purpose statements and ask yourself what is missing. Is information included about the topic? Population? Methods? Concepts or variables? Setting? Outcome? Make appropriate revisions by adding in the missing information.
3. Review the three revised purpose statements and evaluate each according to the evaluation (yes/no questions) checklist. Make appropriate revisions.
4. Identify three professional peers and ask for their constructive feedback on the purpose statements.

_____

_____

_____

_____

_____

_____

_____

_____

### ONLINE/CLASSROOM DISCUSSION

In discussions with your colleagues, share responses to the following:

- In the role of peer reviewer, share your initial purpose statement and review your colleagues' initial purpose statements. After reviewing these, what suggestions would you make to your colleagues for improvements?

## REFERENCES

Cambridge Rindge & Latin School. (2009). *Writing a statement of purpose.* http://www.crlsresearchguide.org/09_writing_state_of_purp.asp

Dusick, D. M. (2014). *Bold educational software: Writing the purpose statement.* http://bold-ed.com/barrc/purpose.htm

Melnyk, B. M., & Fineout-Overholt, E. (2023). *Evidence-based practice in nursing & healthcare: A guide to best practice* (5th ed.). Wolters Kluwer/Lippincott Williams & Wilkins.

Principal Investigators Leader. (2018). *Specific aims & narrative sections: Grab NIH reviewers attention, get your grant funded.* https://www.bu.edu/ctsi/files/2018/01/NIH-Specific-Aims-Narrative-Handouts-GFGW-NI8.pdf

Waldrop, J., & Jennings-Dunlap, J. (2024). Beyond PICO—A new question simplifies the search for evidence. *American Journal of Nursing, 124*(3), 34–37. https://doi.org/10.1097/01.NAJ.0001007676.91191.dd

# 10. Mapping It Out: From Problem to Advanced Clinical Project Plan

## INITIAL THOUGHT

"My project feels like a jigsaw puzzle…how do I make the pieces fit?"

## CHAPTER CONTENT

- Reflective Questions
- Quality Improvement Alert
- Mapping It Out and What That Means
- Project Mapping and the Project Triangle
- Why Use Evidence-Based Quality Improvement Approaches?
- Why Use Evidence Synthesis Plus Approaches?
- Why Use Descriptive Evidence-Generating Approaches?
- Further Considerations for the Project Proposal Map
  - Adding Further Details
  - Is Your Project Feasible?
- Project Mapping: Common Challenges to Avoid
- Summary and Key Points
- Advice From DNP Students
- Practice Scholarship Applications
- Websites for Further Review
- Next Chapter Up
- Online/Classroom Discussion
- Learning Activities
  - To-Do List
  - Possibilities Reflection

## REFLECTIVE QUESTIONS

In Chapter 9, you created a clear purpose statement for your intended project. This chapter guides you in mapping out the big picture of your clinical project. You will be generate ideas for achieving your proposed purpose statement and lay the groundwork for the full project. The following reflective questions organize learning for this chapter. With which of the following are you most confident?

- What strategies for framing evidence-based projects are available?
- How does quality improvement (QI) play into mapping out a project?
- What is your rationale for proposing varied evidence-based projects?
- How will you begin to outline project proposal plans?

Use the Practice Scholarship Applications (at the end of this chapter) to help document your learning from concept to competency, including the relevant American Association of Colleges of Nursing (AACN) *Essentials* (2021).

## QUALITY IMPROVEMENT ALERT

A QI project uses a good systems-based plan for engaging staff and improving patient outcomes. Mapping approaches can be central in planning the full project.

This chapter is about beginning to design (and map) your clinical project proposal. *Designing* and *mapping* mean setting the stage for the project/study. In many cases, the well-designed clinical project can be one step in a change process for improving clinical outcomes. This chapter describes some commonly used approaches for mapping the big picture of your project.

How do you best determine which approach works for your clinical challenges or topic of interest? Clinical projects involve using the best evidence and scholarly methods to help improve patient care. They also involve choosing from various possibilities. Primary questions to address in designing the clinical project map include the following:

1. What is the clinical problem and the clinical unit or population need?
2. What is the current evidence in the literature about the problem?
3. Given the agency/population need and the state of evidence, what will be your project focus or purpose statement? What are the projected outcomes of interest? How will you evaluate what happened?
4. What project approaches will be needed? What tools exist for mapping your project? What type of approach best helps frame the project?

As you consider your project, realize that you have already started to answer these questions in previous chapters. For example, as director of continuing education for a large clinical agency, you note that more staff education on palliative care for your long-term care setting is needed. After completing a systematic literature review, you find that although there is broad information and evidence on palliative care, there is limited information on specific topics such as nutrition and eating issues at the end of life. From your work in this area, you know this is an aspect of concern for both family and staff. In considering this as a clinical project, you have identified a problem, addressed the need in your setting or population, reviewed the current evidence in the literature, considered possible outcomes, and plan to write a purpose statement based on the problem and evidence to guide this.

Now, in this chapter, you will continue to address questions about how to pull all the project pieces together to fit this purpose statement. In some ways, your project is focused for you by determining the level of quality evidence available. If evidence-based protocols are found that can help address your clinical problem and direct practice, an evidence-based QI project may be indicated. If limited evidence exists in your area of concern, descriptive approaches for helping to further generate evidence are likely indicated. If extensive evidence exists and evidence synthesis is needed, that may be a reasonable approach as well.

## MAPPING IT OUT AND WHAT THAT MEANS

Mapping out the clinical project proposal requires you to look at the big picture and sketch out the whole of the project. We have all had experience with maps. In the clinical project, the purpose statement is the project's clear destination. Now the intent is to find the best way, among multiple routes, to reach that destination. This broad path can then guide you in adding further methods detail. The approach for your project proposal (and mapping it out) depends in large part on your organizations's need and your literature review including what evidence is available on your topic.

When writing your project proposal, it helps first to identify a big picture of your plans/methods and then focus on a tight description of a clinical project that can be carried out step by step. This big-picture approach helps you look for your best approach to a needed evidence-based project, as well as potential glitches in the plan that could otherwise be overlooked until it is too late to correct for a meaningful project.

This broad path can then guide you in adding additional methods detail.

## PROJECT MAPPING AND THE PROJECT TRIANGLE

Mapping involves making the points of the project triangle all mesh or intertwine. Recall the need to start with the project purpose and then consider broadly the methods and outcomes. Being prospective in mapping the project helps minimize potential problems by gaining early guidance from faculty and colleagues and clarifying proposal expectations; it provides an opportunity to act in advance to deal with anticipated challenges.

A project map or organizing template is a useful tool since it is much easier to rework a one-page template than to rework a 10- to 20-page proposal. It is a good use of time now, as it saves time later and can reduces the number of problems encountered along the way. Although proposal components are addressed in separate chapters of this book, there is an interplay among them—the components are interrelated and all are needed for completeness and wholeness of the project. The map or organizing template reminds you to pull all of these pieces together and can also help to identify how all the pieces are linked. To build on what you have learned in earlier chapters, it may be helpful to use sample visual tools for brainstorming and problem-solving, including such as concept maps, fishbone diagrams, and other writing tools in preparing for your organizing templates.

Organizing templates provide a type of framework that offers reminders for each project component, often in the format of "filling in the boxes." They can help you begin by providing a starting point to help fill in the boxes (much like putting a puzzle together). Consider using a one-page visual organizer or table and filling in your tentative project pieces there. As you fill in boxes, an additional tool to help fill in this visual organizer can include making use of a problem-solving model, such as the basic nursing process or QI models. A sample project organizing template is provided in Table 10.1 and a simple project example using the Room Safety Scan Project (Bonnel, 2012) is given in Table 10.2.

You have considered the project *necessity* and reviewed evidence-based approaches related to this clinical issue. As noted, before mapping your project plan, you have to consider together your problem topic, agency/population need, and the stage at which the available evidence is currently. This can help direct the project methods and outcomes. Table 10.3 includes common evidence-based approaches to clinical projects.

Considering evidence-based approaches is helpful because you have some initial project direction from the state of the evidence. For example, a concern emerges at work about pain management for patients with dementia. What approaches to a project proposal would be best? Which of the following examples makes the most sense: Implementing an evidence-based protocol (evidence-based QI)? Synthesizing the evidence into a unit protocol (evidence synthesis plus)? Or surveying staff knowledge on pain management and educational needs (evidence generating)? While these might all be possible choices, what you find in the literature about pain management for patients with late-stage dementia can help guide you to one of the following clinical project approaches. See the discussion that follows for these evidence-based approaches.

## TABLE 10.1 EVIDENCE-BASED PROJECT VISUAL ORGANIZER

| | |
|---|---|
| Title of the proposed evidence-based practice project: | Setting: |
| Time frame for completion: | Population of interest: |
| Problem summary: | Current best evidence: |
| Purpose statement: | What conceptual model or theory will guide the project? |
| Proposed project design: Will an intervention be provided? (Is a procedure protocol available or to be developed?) | Major steps of implementation, action items, and target date: |
| What data will be collected? | What tools will be used to collect these data? (What is the quality of the measure?) |
| Who will collect the data? | How will the data-collection methods be systematic and rigorous? |
| How will the data be analyzed? | Potential project strengths/concerns: |

## TABLE 10.2 SAMPLE PROJECT USING ORGANIZING TEMPLATE

| | |
|---|---|
| Tentative title of the proposed EBP project: *The Room Safety Scan* | Setting: 30-bed rehabilitation unit |
| Time frame for completion: *Fall semester* | Population of interest: *Rehab rooms for patients* |
| Problem summary:<br><br>*Patient falls in the clinical setting are a major problem. Literature review suggests intrinsic patient factors are better understood than extrinsic factors.* | Current best evidence:<br><br>*Although literature summarizing intrinsic patient factors leading to falls is evident, limited data are found about the extent of environmental issues leading to falls.* |
| Purpose statement:<br><br>*To raise awareness of fall-safety issues by systematically observing patient rooms for the presence of environmental safety issues.* | What conceptual model or theory will guide the project?<br><br>*Broad systems theory guides attention to structure and process of care to prevent fall outcomes.* |
| Proposed project design: Will an intervention be provided? (Is a procedure protocol available or to be developed?):<br><br>*Descriptive observational project is intended to promote improved quality care.* | Major steps of implementation, action items, and target date<br><br>*No intervention* |
| What data will be collected?<br><br>*Safety factors in 30 occupied patient rooms will be determined.* | What tools will be used to collect these data? (What is the quality of the measure?)<br><br>*A room safety observation checklist will be used. This new tool will be developed from the literature.* |
| Who will collect the data?<br><br>*Project director will collect data over 3 weekends.* | How will the data-collection methods be systematic and rigorous?<br><br>*Peer review to be completed on the observation tool.*<br><br>*A decision trail will be recorded to document the process.* |
| How will the data be analyzed?<br><br>*Descriptive statistics for each safety item and scores as a whole will be reported.* | Potential project strengths/concerns:<br><br>*Gaining team engagement may be a concern.* |

### TABLE 10.3 COMMON EVIDENCE-BASED PROJECT APPROACHES

| Project Type | Descriptor | Example |
| --- | --- | --- |
| Evidence-based quality improvement | Projects that use evidence to solve problems within the contexts of health system | Implementing an already existing evidence-based protocol |
| Evidence synthesis plus | Good evidence exists on your clinical problem in varied articles, but it is not well synthesized | Synthesizing available evidence into a unit protocol |
| Evidence generating | Limited data or research evidence on the problem of interest exists; you might then conduct a project that generates further evidence | Surveying staff knowledge on management of a clinical issue |

## WHY USE EVIDENCE-BASED QUALITY-IMPROVEMENT APPROACHES?

Evidence-based QI projects are often used when a specific need, within a specific context, is identified and extensive evidence syntheses and protocols exist. This involves identifying a problem in your unit and finding an appropriate evidence-based policy in the literature, and then asking: Does a specific evidence-based protocol work in your specified setting?

Perhaps in your literature review, you find the evidence has already been synthesized into a protocol by a respected source. The question becomes: Does the protocol work for your setting and population? For example, you note the aging of your patient population and the increasing incidence of patients with dementia in your unit. The staff seems to lack awareness of how best to communicate with these patients. One project approach could be to further assess and confirm this need for staff improvement, identify and implement an evidence-based communication protocol, and then evaluate the project impact. Both population and system issues can be addressed with these QI-type approaches.

Using a QI framework, these approaches are sometimes considered big-picture frameworks. Some considerations for proposing an evidence-based QI project include the following:

- *Currently available evidence*: High-quality evidence exists in the form of a protocol from a well-respected source.
- *Context*: In concert with the literature, the need exists for this project in your specific population and setting. This need can be reasonably described.
- *Possible methods*: QI models/strategies and procedure implementation and evaluation approaches will be typical.
- *Desired outcomes*: Purpose statement and methods lead to a desired outcome such as adherence to the new protocol and improved nurse comfort using the protocol.
- A summary of an evidence-based QI project relevant to an established staff/provider communication protocol in a unique long-term care setting is provided in Appendix H.

## WHY USE EVIDENCE SYNTHESIS PLUS APPROACHES?

If good evidence exists on your clinical problem but is not well synthesized, you might focus on developing an *evidence synthesis plus* project on this topic. This could lead to a next step, such as a checklist or clinical policy for further testing and evaluation. For purposes of this text, this approach is referred to as an evidence synthesis plus project. Synthesis of the literature involves making the best evidence easily available to health-professional staff. These systematic reviews of the literature can help healthcare providers and staff better understand and use the best clinical evidence to guide clinical decisions.

Especially in new areas of study, the literature synthesis can be a major component of a project. It can lead to developing products such as best evidence checklists, protocols, or decision trees. These projects can serve as a step in translating research to practice that promote safe care delivery and products.

A number of models exist for developing systematic reviews and translating evidence. Melnyk and Fineout-Overholt (2023) describe these models and their similar phases, which include the following:

- Complete the systematic literature review. This involves the steps search, sort, select, and evaluate, and then synthesize common findings.
- Validate the review with an expert's evaluation of the process/content.
- Translate the review for an application product of some type, such as a checklist or protocol.
- Evaluate the product implementation.

Use the following considerations to determine whether the synthesis approach to generating an evidence-based product is reasonable in your situation:

- *Currently available evidence*: You are finding quite a bit of research literature on your focused problem and you are asking questions such as: Is my topic or problem one that has a lot of evidence in the literature? Is it ripe for the synthesis of what is known in nursing or other disciplines? Is it one for which I can access sources of best evidence?
- *Context*: In concert with the literature, the need exists for this project to be performed in a specific population and setting. This need can be reasonably described.
- *Possible methods*: Systematic review and synthesis of the literature, including expert review of the review process and outcomes are considered appropriate. You then synthesize recommendations for practice such as an evidence checklist or a list of needs for further protocol development.
- *Desired outcomes*: Purpose statement and methods lead to a needed synthesis with product developed such as a checklist or protocol for a specific patient population. The product is recommended or tested to identify staff use and satisfaction with the product.

A summary of an evidence synthesis plus project relevant to pediatric patients and surgical anesthesia is provided in Appendix G.

## WHY USE DESCRIPTIVE EVIDENCE-GENERATING APPROACHES?

You have reviewed the evidence and found limited data on your problem or area of interest. Note that this might be considered from a broad evidence perspective (e.g., limited literature or reports from respected national organizations) or could also relate to limited descriptive data specific to your local unit or community.

Since there are limited data or research evidence on the problem or topic of interest, you might then conduct a project that generates further evidence; for example, a project that gains information from families and staff about a specific unit problem. For purposes of this text, this is referred to as a descriptive evidence-generating project. This might include a project such as addressing excess noise and disruption on a clinical unit that prevents needed patient sleep. A project could incorporate asking and observing patients, family, or staff experiences related to this concern.

Or, for example, in relation to an increase in patient falls on the unit, you note that most protocols focus on internal patient factors relevant to falls rather than extrinsic room-safety issues. Further data are needed to help document this problem. You believe that interviews or observations from nursing staff could help generate new data and help raise staff awareness about extrinsic issues relevant to fall prevention. Gaining staff perceptions, completing observations, and reviewing current fall prevention protocols could lead to generating new evidence that could lead to further improvements.

Some considerations for proposing a descriptive evidence-generating project include the following:

- *Currently available evidence*: If you find limited research literature specific to your topic, ask questions such as: Is my topic or problem area one that is new or unique in a selected area? Is this an area that has little evidence available to better understand or guide work with the problem? Is there more need for local data and evidence in the practice world?
- *Context*: In concert with the literature, the need exists for this project in a specific population and setting. This need can be reasonably described.
- *Possible methods*: Many strategies exist to gain basic knowledge/information on a topic relevant to a selected population. Often you will consider basic descriptive study methods for this project. Sometimes the project may be framed as part of a QI project. For example collecting evidence on a given problem, you might use tools such as needs surveys, environmental scans, guided discussion groups, observation tools, or simple interviews or surveys.
- *Desired outcomes*: Purpose statement and methods lead to a needed evidence-generating summary or report that leads to development of a new product or approach.
- A summary of an evidence-generating project from clinician owners of rural clinics is provided in Appendix F.

## FURTHER CONSIDERATIONS FOR THE PROJECT PROPOSAL MAP

Creating a project proposal map is one efficient step to help determine whether your project is feasible. Big-picture project mapping helps to avoid or at least minimize common challenges such as underestimating a project workload, accessing a project setting, and assembling adequate training and resources to carry out the project.

The project map provides guidance to help fill in the project details. It helps answer important project questions such as who, what, when, and where. A broad project map, if clear and appropriate linkages are made, saves one from later problems. Part of this process is clearly aligning the project purpose with the proposed outcomes and methods as depicted in the project triangle. This chapter has laid out a sampling of approaches and methods focusing on concept maps and "filling in the boxes" to help brainstorm and organize the broad project plan. Reviewing a one-page organizing template, along with literature and theory can help you identify where attention is still needed on the project.

## Adding Further Details

Initially, as a work in progress, you will continue detailing your proposed project plan with additional questions. This work in progress moves forward to a detailed plan and serves as a communication tool with colleagues and mentors as well as a guide in writing the proposal. As your project plan matures, questions you will ask include the following:

- What will be the setting?
- Who will be the project participants or subjects?
- What implementation procedures will be used (if any)?
- What specific outcomes are being sought?
- What are best methods for collecting data to evaluate outcomes?
- What will be an appropriate protocol or guidelines to follow for the project?

Fundamental to all is that these questions keep the three points of the project triangle (purpose, methods, and outcomes) aligned.

## Is Your Project Feasible?

The feasibility of your project will further determine your proposal methods. *Feasibility* refers to the project being practical or doable. Consider creating a feasibility checklist for completing the project. Items that can help make a case for feasibility and may also belong in your proposal appendix include

- buy-in from the unit or populations (i.e., is it acceptable to persons involved such as patients, staff, and providers?);
- detailed work plan and timelines (is it effective and efficient in terms of cost and staff time?);
- summary of any needed resources and how they will be obtained;
- summary of needed competencies for completing the project and how they are attained;
- access to people, facilities, and situations, including any needed permissions; and
- procedure approvals from any needed human subjects committees/institutional review boards.

## PROJECT MAPPING: COMMON CHALLENGES TO AVOID

Project mapping and troubleshooting include addressing common practical concerns during the planning phase. Use the following questions to help think about potential issues with your project during project planning.

- Is it the right-sized project—not too large or small?
- Is this the right time and place to address this issue?
- Are you or your team adequately prepared to take on the project?
- Do the points of the project triangle mesh? For example, do the methods, such as data collection, match with the project purpose statement and planned outcomes?
- Are plans too broad or not adequately detailed for others to follow or replicate?
- Are there any political issues or legal considerations in the proposed project setting that might impact project implementation?
- Will the setting be challenging to access?
- Do you (the project director) have adequate background to carry out the project activities?
- Are plans to use selected equipment or resources realistic (Leedy & Ormrod, 2019)?

Also, learn from the experience of DNP students who have preceded you in writing project proposals; see the box titled Advice From DNP Students.

### ADVICE FROM DNP STUDENTS

**Project Mapping**

Think about the big picture.

- The proposal is like a huge jigsaw puzzle. Everything has to fit perfectly together or it does not work. Changing even a small study component can result in a totally different focus for a project.

Diagram, in the most basic and simple format, what needs to happen.

- I am learning how to take a project idea and attempt to distill it down to the most basic elements for the project.

Use your initial work to generate more questions.

- The more I read, the more questions I have.

Discuss with others.

- Interaction with others is helpful in that it highlights aspects of the project that you might not have thought about.
- Learning from my colleagues as they developed their project ideas was captivating.

> **PRACTICE SCHOLARSHIP APPLICATIONS**
>
> Consider your competency documentation plans. How will your project address select *Essentials*? Consider additions to your project notebook as you complete the following.
>
> - *Concepts to competence*: Review questions from the beginning of this chapter and self-assess on your progress. Appreciate your accomplishments in project mapping, as documented in your project notebook.
> - *Essentials*: Review advanced level competencies and subcompetencies for the Knowledge for Nursing Practice, Scholarship for Nursing Practice, and Quality and Safety *Essentials* domains and reflect on how they relate to your clinical project.
> - *Project notebook*: Complete a one-page map of your project plans. Include a written reflection that considers potential challenges and successes of the plan.

## SUMMARY AND KEY POINTS

Mapping out the big picture of your project helps maintain the desired direction. You have identified your problem and the literature surrounding this problem. You have started to address the context or setting and population issues. Now, considering the project triangle, what approach seems the best match? As your project ideas come together, use techniques from this chapter to map out plans that can guide your project. Points to recall from this chapter include the following:

- Mapping a project means to look at the big picture of your project in terms of a selected pathway or approach. This broad path can then guide you in adding additional methods detail.
- Project mapping includes using the project triangle, and tools such as, concept maps, and organizing templates to diagram the big picture.
- Templates that flow from the project triangle provide guidance in beginning to fill in project details.
- In addition to clinical unit or population need, the state of the evidence related to your project topic helps guide you in choosing a clinical project pathway or approach. Common choices include an evidence-based QI project, an evidence synthesis plus pathway, or descriptive evidence-generating approach.

## WEBSITES FOR FURTHER REVIEW

Mapping ideas can be gained by reviewing resources at select websites such as national reports from the National Academy of Sciences and the Agency for Healthcare Research and Quality (AHRQ). Ideas for small-scale projects might be gained from the following as well as from similar national reports.

- *Making Eye Health a Population Health Imperative: Vision for Tomorrow*:

    www.nap.edu/catalog/23471/making-eye-health-a-population-health-imperative-vision-for-tomorrow
- *AHRQ Fall Prevention Toolkit*:

    www.ahrq.gov/sites/default/files/publications/files/fallpxtoolkit.pdf

## NEXT CHAPTER UP

As discussed in this chapter, you are working on a big-picture map of your project proposal. The next chapter helps add the additional detail of more specific methods to use. In general, this includes data-collection tools (often from research or QI methods) and strategies that assist in implementing and evaluating your project. Remember that although components of each of the proposal chapters are addressed separately, there is an interplay among all components; each piece is needed to create a complete, cohesive project.

> **ONLINE/CLASSROOM DISCUSSION**
>
> Share your one-page project map with your colleagues. Use this as a time to share feedback and ideas related to shared projects.

## LEARNING ACTIVITIES

### To-Do List

1. Finalize the literature review for best evidence on your topic of interest.
2. Address staff/unit/population need for the proposed plan.
3. Determine the type and quality of literature that exists for your problem of interest.
4. Create a possibilities reflection (see the following learning activity).
5. Begin mapping your plan through a project template.

### Possibilities Reflection

Reflective writing can often help better determine a map of possibilities for detailing a project related to a specific problem/topic. Reflecting on possibilities might include the following:

- To learn more about my problem/topic, I might observe the following activities/situations: _____ _____.

- I might talk to the following people: _____ _____.

- I might review the following documents/resources: _____ _____.

- Various ways to address this problem/topic from a project-methods perspective would include: _____ _____.

- The most reasonable way to address this problem/topic from a project-methods perspective would be: _____ _____.

## REFERENCES

Bonnel, M. (2012). *The room safety scan project*. Unpublished manuscript. Department of Nursing, Fort Hays State University.

Leedy, P., & Ormrod, J. (2019). *Practical research: Planning and design* (12th ed.). Pearson.

Melnyk, B. M., & Fineout-Overholt, E. (2023). *Evidence-based practice in nursing & healthcare: A guide to best practice* (5th ed.). Wolters Kluwer/Lippincott Williams & Wilkins.

# 11. Writing the Method Section: Organizing the Advanced Clinical Project Proposal

## INITIAL THOUGHT

"The method section is in some ways like a cookbook. It has to be as specific as a recipe so that others can follow what you have done."

## CHAPTER CONTENT

- Reflective Questions
- Quality Improvement Alert
- The Importance of the Method Section
- Focusing the Project Methods
  - Methods for Gaining Data: The Project Triangle
- Data Collection: Which Methods Will Gain the Desired Evaluation Data?
- Qualitative and Quantitative Paradigms (And Why They Matter)
  - Qualitative Context: Issues to Consider
  - Quantitative Context: Issues to Consider
- Strategies for Collecting/Gaining Data
  - Interviews and Surveys
    - Written Surveys
    - Planning for Interviews or Surveys
  - Observations
  - Record or Document Reviews
- Additional Comments on Data Collection
- Data-Collection Examples Using the Project Triangle
  - Descriptive Evidence Generation
  - Evidence-Based Quality Improvement
- Setting and Sample Considerations for Your Proposal
  - Describe the Setting Clearly
  - Describe Population and Sampling Choices Clearly
- So, Which Approaches Do You Use for the Proposal?
- Common Approaches to Writing Up the Methods
- Advice From DNP Students
- Practice Scholarship Applications
- Summary and Key Points
- Websites for Further Review
- Next Chapter Up
- Online/Classroom Discussion
- Learning Activities
  - Reflecting Further on Your Project Plans
  - Pulling the Method Section Together in Your Proposal
  - To-Do List

## REFLECTIVE QUESTIONS

In Chapter 10, you considered the importance of mapping out broad plans for your proposal. The following reflective questions help you consider development of your method section and organize learning for this chapter. With which of the following are you most confident?

- What makes detailing proposal methods important?
- What specific methods are addressed in the proposal?
- What specific approaches could work for your project?
- Will the proposed methods produce the outcomes you seek?

Use the Practice Scholarship Applications (at the end of this chapter) to help document your learning from concept to competency, including relevant American Association of Colleges of Nursing (AACN) *Essentials* (2021).

## QUALITY IMPROVEMENT ALERT

The method section states what you will do, where, and with whom in your quality improvement (QI) project, so provide specific steps that anyone could easily follow.

## THE IMPORTANCE OF THE METHOD SECTION

This chapter helps identify the big picture regarding QI and/or research methods for your project. A function of the method section is to address what you plan to do and why you plan to do it. The method section describes the process that will be used to gain the project product or outcomes. If you are proposing either an evidence-based QI approach or a descriptive evidence-generating approach for your project, the following elements need to be described:

- *Setting*: Specify elements of the specific setting in your project, providing sufficient detail of the project context (so that others are aware of similarities or differences from their own settings).
- *Population*: Specify the population you will work with or study, giving at least a broad description of expected participants.
- *If intervention is to be used*: Describe the intervention and its component parts in enough detail that others could reproduce it; outline initial plans for how the intervention is to be implemented.
- *Data collection*: Describe the specific data-collection plan.

If you are choosing an *evidence synthesis plus* process, your approach will be a bit different. Because the initial focus in the evidence synthesis plus project is the literature review, further planning points will depend on your "plus." As indicated, this may relate to using the evidence synthesis to develop checklists to be used for chart review, specific clinical protocol development from the evidence, or other QI approaches.

Writing a project proposal incorporates many components. The key in aligning these components is the project triangle. This chapter focuses on the methods point of the triangle and helps to address "how to do the methods."

## FOCUSING THE PROJECT METHODS

Project methods will vary depending on the project approach you choose. Let's say you are working with patients with Parkinson disease (PD) and want to develop a project related to support groups for those patients. In this example, the assessment of your population, potential settings, and the literature suggest the benefit of a descriptive evidence-generating project (you will learn more about the perspectives of these individuals).

In a second example, if you had a strong evidence base or protocol for a needed topic in your clinical setting, perhaps swallowing problems in patients with late-stage PD, you might decide to share a new protocol, a type of intervention, with your staff using an evidence-based QI approach. When intervention is to be used in your project, you will incorporate the following:

- Address the context factors for your project. This includes place factors (the healthcare practice context) and people factors (patient-specific variables and staff type/amount of staffing) that are the background for the intervention protocol.
- Outline initial plans for how the intervention is to be implemented.
- Describe the intervention and its component parts in sufficient detail so that others can reproduce it.
- Address components to include in your planning, such as who will implement the intervention (individuals or multiple people) and their qualifications (or the methods needed to train them)?
- Consider any issues concerning internal validity of the project intervention and plans for monitoring the fidelity of the intervention and describe this as thoroughly as possible.
- Implement and evaluate the protocol, which will also include monitoring data-collection plans such as the Standards for Quality Improvement Reporting Excellence (2015). This QI document provides further guidance.

As you read through this chapter, continue to refer to the text in Box 11.1 and think about the initial challenges presented in project planning. Note similarities and differences between these approaches and the one you are working on.

### BOX 11.1 Methods Questions: Parkinson Disease Online Support Group Example

If you are working with patients with Parkinson disease (PD) and are concerned about their emotional support issues, what are some of the problems/issues that come to mind? What are some potential responses by healthcare providers? What might lead to a project to help address identified needs? Your response, of course, is to head to the literature to gain answers. You will have to first review the literature to determine the best evidence for support groups as a resource. This will include a review of evidence specifically for patients with PD. What questions come to mind for the need you have identified and the best type of project methods?

- Based on the evidence available, should your project implement and evaluate support groups or are further questions raised? What do you still need to know?
- Does your evidence address the changing needs of patients who are progressing through the disease? Does the literature cover all disease stages, or are there special needs for patients with later stages of the disease versus early stages of the disease?
- Does your literature address the setting or context for support groups? Does the literature address advancing PD and online versus face-to-face group strategies/challenges?
- If you find there is little evidence in the literature on PD patients and support group issues, what are your options for framing a project? Would you be more likely to work with early stage or later stage patients? Would you be more likely to consider a descriptive project, gaining patient perspectives about the need for and benefits (or challenges) of support groups, or implement and evaluate a protocol for a specific type of support group? How will you consider setting, populations, intervention potential, and data collection?

## Methods for Gaining Data: The Project Triangle

Making the methods choices fit or align with the project purpose and desired project outcomes is the goal. Recall the project triangle (see Appendix A), in which the purpose, methods, and outcomes represent the three triangle points. Any inconsistency among the three will make the triangle fall apart (as the three lines won't match up into the shape of a triangle). In going back to the project triangle, your project purpose (based on the chosen clinical problem and current evidence found in the literature) also dictates the types of methods needed for a complete/quality project. Ask: What has the purpose statement promised? What are the intended outcomes? This guides choices for data collection. For example, when you plan to collect project data, you will be making choices about interviews, surveys, observations, document reviews, or some combination thereof.

The purpose statement provides the basis for a descriptive evidence-generating project, an evidence synthesizing plus project, or an evidence-based QI-type project. Again, there needs to be consistency among the purpose, methods, and outcomes you choose for your project.

## DATA COLLECTION: WHICH METHODS WILL GAIN THE DESIRED EVALUATION DATA?

Data-collection plans provide one of the most interesting parts of the project proposal. It is here that you devise plans to organize information, implement processes, and collect evidence specific to your project outcomes. Central to clinical scholarship (i.e., to make sure you have good data to share), you need good methods for data collection. Approaches to be considered include (a) interview/survey, (b) observations, and (c) document or electronic record reviews. A reminder of these approaches, from your previous coursework, is provided in quick summary format in Table 11.1.

Once broad choices are made, you will prepare a more detailed plan (negotiating the best tools and approaches) while keeping in mind the practical resources available; these are all considerations in planning your methods. You want to use the best methods possible to get the best results since even one weak piece can lead to a weak project. Adding detail to the data-collection methods is further described via qualitative and quantitative paradigms.

## QUALITATIVE AND QUANTITATIVE PARADIGMS (AND WHY THEY MATTER)

How will you begin to further detail the methods? The project purpose you choose influences the methods you use. For example, if your purpose is to generate evidence on a new clinical challenge, then you might choose either a qualitative

| TABLE 11.1 DATA-COLLECTION TOOLS | | |
|---|---|---|
| Tool | Sample Approaches | Your Examples: |
| Surveys | Face-to-face written survey<br>E-mail survey<br>Electronic survey | |
| Interviews | Face-to-face<br>Group-guided discussions | |
| Observations | Clinical labs<br>Clinical settings<br>Public settings | |
| Record reviews | Electronic chart reviews<br>Agency document reviews (often web based) | |

or quantitative survey approach to gain data about that challenge. As you will note, within the qualitative or quantitative paradigms, various common data-collection methods include interviews, surveys, observations, or document reviews. The paradigm you choose should guide the more specific methods chosen. For example, if the qualitative approach is chosen, then the qualitative theme typically guides the plan throughout its duration. In other words, written surveys or interview prompts are primarily open ended or use a basic descriptive format. If quantitative approaches are chosen, you would use more structured surveys or interview approaches with numeric responses/rating scales.

The following paragraphs first consider qualitative versus quantitative approaches for methods choices. Then common tools used within both qualitative and quantitative paradigms (interviews, surveys, observations, and document reviews) are discussed. Again, Table 11.1 provides sample approaches to using various common data-collection methods.

## Qualitative Context: Issues to Consider

The qualitative paradigm considers the world through a lens of openness and complexity. The value of broad, open-ended questions directed by qualitative paradigms includes gaining perspectives from the subject about their perceived knowledge, attitudes, or behaviors. Qualitative methods typically include gaining some type of word data, as opposed to numeric data. Content analysis for common themes is typically used with themes summarizing the data obtained.

- Qualitative methods provide a beginning tool kit for gaining data that can be authentic and meaningful. Well-known qualitative tools, such as broad interview questions and observations, bring real-world experiences to life through the written word and provide descriptive richness for data sharing.

- Qualitative data can serve as the basic descriptive data for sharing or developing future projects. Qualitative methods capture word themes that convey experiences in a richer texture than quantitative numbers alone.
- Benefits of qualitative methods include gaining subjects' true understandings from their own perspectives, whereby a depth of understanding missing from numerical summaries can be gained. Typically, a small sample size will be beneficial in learning about others' experiences. For example, if you wanted to gain needs assessment data on those in a new role such as NICU nurses, you might interview those individuals to better understand challenges. Sample approaches include broad open-ended *interviews* or *surveys*, either with individuals or with groups.
- Broad observation guides for a specific setting or population can also be used with qualitative approaches. They provide, for example, opportunities to make broad observations such as "walk-throughs" or windshield surveys of new or unique settings. Theories or models from community or public health or organizational leadership coursework can provide examples for strategies to organize these initial observations.
- Challenges to qualitative approaches include the small sample sizes used, which often limit the ability to generalize the findings. These are typically descriptive projects that do not focus on testing interventions. They are often used for evidence-generating descriptive projects, including needs assessments. They are also used to gain qualitative perspectives in evaluative projects.

## Quantitative Context: Issues to Consider

The quantitative paradigm is considered to be focused and deterministic; often this approach is compared to a closed system. Quantitative approaches are used to capture and summarize knowledge, attitudes, or behaviors numerically. This involves using tools to gain numerical data representing these qualities (as opposed to word data generated in the qualitative approach).

- These tools provide an opportunity to gain data that can help one understand the numerical qualities of an attribute. Surveys and other tools for observation and document review help specify through numbers what is going on or enable the researcher to make comparisons.
- Quantitative approaches can also help describe and make a compelling case for projects in early descriptive stages, including large needs assessments. Quantitative methods capture numeric summaries that promote ease of comparison and help summarize large groups of responses more easily than qualitative themes.
- A quantitative approach is often useful in data collection for projects, such as evidence-based QI projects, that evaluate a new protocol.
- Challenges to this method include finding measures or survey instruments that truly capture the concepts being studied. Quantitative approaches lose the richness of descriptive themes gained with qualitative methods but have the benefit of more easily conveying or comparing numerical data about diverse groups. Along with the need for the instrument to measure what you intend (validity), the instrument must also be able to measure that concept accurately and repeatedly (reliability).

Note that sometimes qualitative and quantitative approaches are mixed in the same project in attempts to gain the benefits of each approach. Further reading in research texts can provide more direction on these approaches.

## STRATEGIES FOR COLLECTING/GAINING DATA

As noted, qualitative and quantitative paradigms provide the broad context or background assumptions for the choices you make in gaining data. These paradigms set the stage for the more detailed data-collection plan to learn about the problem or topic of interest. How many ways are there to collect data? To keep things simple, broad approaches of interview and survey, observation, and record review (e.g., charts or electronic health records [EHRs]) need to be discussed in your proposal. Further choices and details then need to be added to each. Information about these common tools for gaining project data follows.

### Interviews and Surveys

Interviews and surveys provide an opportunity to gain information about people's knowledge, attitudes, or perceived behaviors. Interview guides and surveys can be developed from either qualitative or quantitative perspectives. Qualitative methods more typically use open-ended questions with verbal responses. Quantitative approaches typically use closed-ended questions that seek some type of response with numerical coding potential.

- *Face-to-face individual interviews*: These provide an opportunity to converse with an individual about a specific topic, typically to gain others' perceptions. They include the value of engaging in nonverbal communication about the topic/questions. Opportunities to extend questions and generate follow-up responses to questions that emerge can be valuable.
- *Face-to-face group interviews*: These provide the benefit of gaining individuals' thoughts on a topic. They also provide further opportunities to stimulate ideas from others with brainstorming-type approaches to gain ideas/topics individuals may not have thought to share. Challenges may be to make sure the investigator

receives a true opinion versus "group think." In research studies, a more detailed approach to group interviews is referred to as a *focus group*.

## Written Surveys

Written surveys can be designed for paper-and-pencil or electronic formats. They provide the opportunity to learn from others' knowledge or experience related to a topic. They can be easy to administer, but a disadvantage they share is they offer no opportunity to follow up or clarify why the individual responded as they did. The intent is for participants to interpret and respond as the investigator intends. Ideally, these are well-tested tools with strong reliability and validity. If the tools are new, piloting and evaluation work are required.

## Planning for Interviews or Surveys

When considering interviews or surveys, basic questions include: Are well-developed tools available? Are these appropriate qualitative or quantitative approaches? Do they define the concepts of interest in the same way as your project does? Tool descriptions are further addressed in Chapters 12 and 13.

You also need to plan and be very specific in your proposal regarding the actual strategies you will use in completing the interviews or surveys. For example, what will be the context or setting for the written or face-to-face data collection? Where will this happen? Will there be privacy if this is a sensitive subject? Will there be an opportunity to collect data during a scheduled clinic waiting time or before a class? How will participants return these forms to you? As noted, use of online surveys is another possibility. They add to the speed of data collection as long as participants can easily access the survey and have the motivation to complete it.

## Observations

Observation allows the opportunity to view activities in natural settings (Warren & Karner, 2014) and to learn new information or confirm concepts and processes. Observation has value when learning about situations, behaviors, and competencies. Observing classrooms or clinical agencies, the investigator learns about roles, practices, and strategies of people observed and also gains information about the setting's structure and processes. Observations may be used less frequently than surveys and interviews, but they are valuable in learning about real-life behaviors.

Specifying or mapping out and documenting a plan that includes time or event factors to observe allows better opportunity to capture what is intended. For example, if you are interested in socialization among residents in a long-term group activity room, you may decide to use a very detailed plan for scheduled activity observations, including length of time for observation, the observer's role, and specific schedule of observations. Observation data can also be collected in more structured settings like simulation skills labs; for example, staff nurses' experiences in a simulation lab to seek concepts related to ethical decision-making as part of the simulation. Clinical lab observations also provide opportunities related to staff development and competency assessment.

## Record or Document Reviews

A common data-collection strategy, especially in QI, is chart reviews. This is a nonintrusive strategy for collecting data. Formerly this was done on hard copies of charts; EHRs have now emerged.

EHRs have changed the way chart reviews are done and provide many advantages. The speed of review is one of these. Fairly rapidly, these tools provide collections of data that would have taken hours to access and review in the past. It is important to remember that just as chart-review projects included a data-collection sheet, the electronic equivalent of this sheet is still required. Asking random questions about the data will not lead to a good analysis. You need to give thought to how you structure your electronic data-collection guide.

Chart reviews can also provide challenges to data collection. Challenges or disadvantages to EHRs and other forms of record review include that the clinician/researcher has no control over the data collected. For example, if you are reviewing care processes, there may be inaccuracies in the recording; that is, something might have actually been done but not charted. Or, if physiologic measures, such as blood pressures, are gained (usually fairly strong credible measures), there is no control over the protocol used in gaining these measures. Also, there is no ability to ask further questions about missing data.

Advantages or benefits of EHR data include reasonable access to clinical data that can help answer, in particular, QI questions. Large electronic databases, such as the National Database of Nursing Quality Indicators, also exist and may be valuable in collecting meaningful data for specified project purposes.

## ADDITIONAL COMMENTS ON DATA COLLECTION

Again, for each data-collection method (interview, survey, observation, and record review), there are many variations related to the structure of items. This includes, for example, highly structured questions through the quantitative paradigm as well as the open-ended structure of questions guided by the qualitative paradigm. In some cases, diverse methods can also be combined in useful/appropriate ways, providing a type of triangulation. A good research text can provide further detail to guide additional decisions. With all cases of data collection, it is necessary to address appropriate human subjects and Health Insurance Portability and Accountability Act guidelines as required. This is discussed in Chapter 14.

Refer again to Table 11.1, which provides sample approaches to using these common data-collection tools. Each of these tools can be considered from both qualitative and quantitative perspectives. As you review, consider how many ways there are to use each of these. Have fun with this and consider also how each might (or might not) be relevant to the project you are planning.

## DATA-COLLECTION EXAMPLES USING THE PROJECT TRIANGLE

Remember that whatever method you choose must allow alignment of the points of the project triangle. Purpose, methods, and outcomes need to support each other. Project triangle examples, specific to evidence-generating and evidence-testing methods, follow.

### Descriptive Evidence Generation

- *Purpose*: To determine need for an onsite health clinic at a large assisted-living setting.
- *Methods*: Qualitative observations of setting (people and place factors) and qualitative interviews with staff/residents about current processes and additional need for healthcare.
- *Seeking outcomes*: Needs assessment report that summarizes planning needs for an onsite clinic.

### Evidence-Based Quality Improvement

- *Purpose*: To determine success of a new evidence-based discharge protocol for patients with congestive heart failure.
- *Methods*: Qualitative/quantitative survey of patients and their family members on readiness for discharge; guided discussion with staff on challenges/strategies for using the protocol.
- *Seeking outcomes*: Documentation of successful protocol or needed improvements.

## SETTING AND SAMPLE CONSIDERATIONS FOR YOUR PROPOSAL

Clearly identifying in your proposal the setting and the population your project will study is key to helping your reader gain context. Consider the following setting and population issues as you make your plans and write up the method section.

### Describe the Setting Clearly

To describe the setting, you will describe elements of the specific setting in your project. For example, if you want to consider the benefits of educational gaming as a strategy for a clinical education-related problem in a large healthcare system, the education protocol could be placed in the context of all staff education: health professions education, nursing-student education, or nursing-staff development education. It could also be placed in the frame of one clinical unit, a large healthcare system, or systems across a state or the country. Clearly framing your setting (and sample) helps focus your project.

To describe this context or setting for your project, you might first create a big-picture description or "systems" perspective of the overall setting and then fill in the parts/details such as the relevant people factors, place factors, and process factors related to the issue or topic. For example, in a study of a particular long-term care unit, you might identify the types of rooms, the number of people in the setting, common unit activities, and other factors relevant to your project. You might address what makes this unit similar or different from others.

### Describe Population and Sampling Choices Clearly

In research courses, you discussed the differences between populations (the larger context of potential participants) and samples (specific participants). Now consider the different options in sampling choices and make complementary choices to match your project methods. For example, in qualitative projects, typically the convenience sample dominates. In early descriptive stages of the study, a small $N$ is considered acceptable. Smaller numbers can still provide important descriptive information to help understand a topic or learn about populations' needs. For example, if you are asking rural nurses about challenges and approaches they use to best support patients in settings with scant resources, a sample size of 10 could provide good beginning descriptive data. A qualitative project can help describe and make a compelling initial case relevant to a clinical problem.

Quantitative projects tend to be more interested in using a sample that is representative of the population in question so, in general, samples have larger numbers so that they are more representative of the population of interest. Assumptions for quantitative statistics, for example, indicate at least an $N$ of 30 to represent the population. Random sampling provides value in meeting assumptions for more sophisticated statistical procedures. Further discussion about quantitative statistics required for a project analysis is presented in Chapter 13.

How will your sampling choices relate to your projected outcomes and analyses? These choices play a major role in determining to whom the results of your project may be relevant. This applies, for example, if you want to make the case that your results have implications beyond your population sample and setting; in other words, generalizing findings to another population or setting. In many clinical projects, you will describe as clearly as possible your methods and findings, but not have an adequate sample size or adequate control of external variables to generalize these findings. If that is the case, your detailed project can still be useful to others who may wish to replicate your project and see whether similar outcomes are gained in their setting.

Making a good sampling choice involves knowing your project plan and the strengths and weaknesses of varied sampling approaches. In addition, it is critical to consider whether the preferred approach is actually doable. Sometimes, there are trade-offs between what is preferred and what is doable; therefore, you, as the project director, must make the case for why you make the choices you make. Ask yourself the following questions about potential sampling in your project:

- Is the population clearly defined? Is the population accessible?
- Are choices of convenience or random sampling justified?
- Are sampling procedures sufficiently detailed for replication?
- Are sampling choices appropriate to the project purpose statement?

For example, as you address your project plans, consider this chapter's case examples related to interests with support groups for patients with PD (see Box 11.1). Varied considerations are needed to identify your population and ultimately your sample. Some of the descriptive components and questions related to the population of study would include the following:

- Who makes up the broad population of patients with PD in your region of interest?
- Who makes up the accessible population? Are there currently groups that involve patients in the beginning, middle, or late stages of the disease?
- Will these individuals be found in groups that are online or face-to-face?
- Do the groups involve caregivers, families, or patients only or a mix? Are there other unique population factors that should be considered; for example, younger versus older patients?

Making informed choices about potential participants for data collection is an important proposal component. Will you describe an entire population or selected subgroups? What populations (such as community, state, or regional populations or clinical unit entities) will provide you the information you need?

## SO, WHICH APPROACHES DO YOU USE FOR THE PROPOSAL?

This chapter talks broadly about methods. But which methods you choose will relate most closely to the type of clinical project design you focus on. As you consider your topic, think back to Box 11.1 and any similarities it may have to the PD support group example. As described in Chapter 10, selected ways to use the best evidence for projects include the following:

- *Evidence synthesis plus*: Does literature/evidence exist about support groups that have not been synthesized for patients with PD? Would evidence lead to protocols for online groups or face-to-face groups? These could be possibilities for your project.
- *Evidence-based QI*: Does evidence exist in the form of a protocol for chronic care support groups that could be evaluated specifically for PD? Could the protocol be further validated as successful by participants or providers? These could be possibilities for your project.
- *Descriptive evidence generation*: Is more evidence needed related to specific concerns about groups for patients with PD? Could you ask clients in support groups their opinions? Could you ask clinical providers their opinions? Would possibilities exist for using interviews or surveys to gain further data? These could be possibilities for your project.

Again, once the literature has been evaluated and a purpose statement determined, your project purpose will guide the methods you use. Within those larger paradigms of qualitative approaches and quantitative approaches, choices about surveys, interviews, observation, or document review will also be considered. Begin to map out the project triangle with appropriate methods to develop proposal plans. Guidance for the appropriate use of methods for the type of project you are conducting is developed with a mentor.

## COMMON APPROACHES TO WRITING UP THE METHODS

Where and how does the method section fit in the proposal? Scholarly proposals are typically arranged in sections that first include introductory materials, then the review of the literature, and third, the detailed method section. Within the method section, the common scholarly "parts" (or subsections, often with headings) noted in the following list can help organize your project methods. Specifically describe in your plan the following as part of your method section:

- *Setting*: Specify elements of the specific setting in your project.
- *Population/sampling*: How is the population defined (inclusion/exclusion criteria)?

- *Sampling*: Specify your project population and provide at least a broad description of expected project participants.
- *Specific project implementation plans and evaluation methods*: Describe any intervention or procedure in fine detail. These strategies should be described in enough specific detail so that others (in their own unique settings) could replicate the interventions or procedures you use.

Creating a table of contents can serve as a helpful guide in organizing key components of the method section. If you are in school as you complete your project, the school often has set guidelines for the specific headings to be used for the proposal. If you are in a clinical agency with specific criteria to be addressed before submission to the human subjects committee, that criteria need to be addressed as well. If yours is a clinical proposal to seek funding, funding agencies typically outline specified categories to be addressed. Turning these latter guidelines into headings when possible helps the reader and typically improves the quality of the product. As previously noted, an abstract or two-page draft of your plan can keep the proposal tightly packaged for discussions and decision-making by team members.

Also learn from the experience of DNP students who have preceded you in developing project proposals. Their advice is presented in the Advice From DNP Students box.

## SUMMARY AND KEY POINTS

This chapter talks broadly about methods and choices for use in clinical project proposals. Qualitative and quantitative paradigms provide background for common data-collection choices of interviews, surveys, observations, and record reviews. The methods you choose will relate to the purpose and outcomes on which you plan to focus. As noted, there are multiple approaches to these topics. Various choices keep clinical projects interesting and echo the importance of identifying early on exactly what you need and want to do. Points to recall from this chapter include the following:

- Your project method section should be specific enough that others can reproduce them. The method section gives you direction and allows others to know your project plan. Some describe this as being as specific as a protocol or "recipe" that others could follow.
- Focusing the project methods includes paying attention to context. For example, clearly describing the setting and clearly describing sampling choices are key points of your proposal.
- Method section choices need to fit with the project purpose and desired project outcomes. Consider points of the project triangle when planning how to gain

### ADVICE FROM DNP STUDENTS

**Methods**

Think about putting together the pieces of the proposal puzzle.
- It is certainly like searching for detail after detail to fit each piece together.
- In retrospect, I should have spent more time looking for and reviewing similar projects to guide my thought process.

Go back to your textbooks.
- Once you have a plan in mind, reexamine what your research text says about your particular plans (e.g., if you plan to use a descriptive survey, read more about that).

Focus on your specific methods.
- Try to think methodically about each and every step for data collection.
- While reading, everything seems important to know, understand, and apply. Focus on the chapters or concepts that should get most of the attention.

Structure the method section.
- Learn how to structure the method section of a project proposal and remember the importance of being complete and thorough.

Be clear in your write-up of the method section.
- When writing a method section, what seems clear the first several times you write out the details, probably isn't. Every time I came back to read my method section I realized it wasn't as clear as it seemed when I looked at it the time before. I was still tweaking the final product up until the moment I submitted the proposal. The devil is truly in the details.

### PRACTICE SCHOLARSHIP APPLICATIONS

Consider your competency documentation plans. How will your project address select *Essentials*? Consider additions to your project notebook as you complete the following:

- *Concepts to competence*: Think about your knowledge of methods. What methods best fit your project purpose and desired outcomes? Think about and justify the methods you've selected for your clinical project.
- *Essentials*: Review advanced level competencies and subcompetencies for the Knowledge for Nursing Practice and Scholarship for the Nursing Discipline *Essential* domains. Reflect on how they relate to your clinical project methods.
- *Project notebook*: Include a one-page written reflection that addresses your project's methods, including setting, population/sample, intervention plans for QI, data collection plans, and evaluation data.

evaluative project data. Review the project triangle to ensure all components of your plan are covered and fit together.

- Qualitative and quantitative paradigms provide background for methods choices.
  - Issues to consider when using a qualitative context typically include descriptive methods and a smaller sample size.
  - Issues to consider when using a quantitative context typically include a larger sample size and more structured numerical data-collection methods.
- Project evaluation data can be gained through selected approaches with broad categories, including interviews, surveys, record or document reviews, and observations as methods for data collection. There are pros and cons to use of each.
- Writing up the method section includes paying attention to detail.

## WEBSITES FOR FURTHER REVIEW

When planning a method section, keep returning to your project purpose. Examples of resources that offer more ideas for method sections can be seen by reviewing online examples and resources at select websites. See examples at the following websites:

- *Qualitative resources*:
  https://researchmethod.net/qualitative-research/
- *Quantitative evaluation tools and instruments*:
  https://informalscience.org/projects/evaluation-instruments/

Ideas for project protocols can also be gained by reviewing resources such as those provided by the National Academy of Sciences. Ideas for small-scale projects might be gained from these and similar national reports.

- *Families Caring for an Aging America* (this National Academy of Sciences report addresses family needs and challenges related to caregiving, as well as synthesizing successful interventions and outcomes):
  https://nap.nationalacademies.org/catalog/23606/families-caring-for-an-aging-america

## NEXT CHAPTER UP

As you consider approaches to data collection, you are also thinking ahead as to how you will get credible data. You will consider strategies for data collection that promote confidence in the tools chosen for your project and help to ensure that the resultant findings are reliable and valid.

### ONLINE/CLASSROOM DISCUSSION

In discussions with your colleagues, based on the readings, address the following case study.

*Case study*: In your hospital, you want to implement and evaluate an evidence-based strategy for communication tips to prevent agitated behaviors in patients with dementia.

What strategies could you suggest to enhance sampling and project methods and approaches for the following:

- Begin project roll-out with a large hospital-wide program? Or pilot/evaluate on one specific clinical unit? Other choices?
- Who would you collect outcome data from? What type of data would you collect? What would be your methods for data collection?
- How could you set up this plan using the points of the project triangle (purpose, methods, and outcomes)?

## LEARNING ACTIVITIES

### Reflecting Further on Your Project Plans

- At this point, what seems to be reasonable and might work for the plan you are considering?
- What other options might also work?
- Address the pros and cons of each of your ideas. What will best meet your planned purpose? What will work best given your context and experience?

### Pulling the Method Section Together in Your Proposal

If you are collecting data for your clinical project, does your proposal address each of the following?

- Does it have methods that fit the project purpose and proposed outcomes?
- Does it provide a description of the population and a strategy for sampling?
- Does it provide specific project implementation plans and evaluation?
- Does it specify procedures for data collection?
- What is its timeline?
- Have you verified resource accessibility?
- Have you resolved any human subjects and institutional review board issues?

### To-Do List

1. Complete further reading related to specific approaches you would like to use in your project. Look at examples

of other projects that have been completed using similar methods.
2. Consider how you will best access the people or physical resources needed to complete your project.
3. Consider the "so what" or "why this is important" factors related to your proposed plans.

## REFERENCES

Standards for Quality Improvement Reporting Excellence. (2015). *Revised standards for quality improvement reporting excellence, SQUIRE 2.0.* http://www.squire-statement.org/index.cfm?fuseaction=Page.ViewPage&PageID=471

Warren, C., & Karner, T. (2014). *Discovering qualitative methods: Field research, interviews, and analysis* (3rd ed.). Oxford University Press.

# 12. Gaining Credible Clinical Project Data: Being Systematic and Objective

## INITIAL THOUGHT

"You are going to do a lot of work for your project, so you really want it to be good."

## CHAPTER CONTENT

- Reflective Questions
- Quality Improvement Alert
- Providing a Detailed Plan for Data Collection
  - With Your Clinical Project in Mind
- Describing Credible/Trustworthy Tools
  - Share a Thorough Description
  - Share Reliability and Validity
  - Describe Related Credibility Issues
  - Describe the Protocol Procedure for Data Collection
  - Pilot Test of Tools and Procedures
- Other Considerations
  - The Setting
  - Data Organization
  - Storing Data
  - Data-Collection Timeline
  - Technology and Data Collection
- Further Challenges
  - Instrument Development
  - Project Internal Validity
- Advice From DNP Students
- Practice Scholarship Applications
- Summary and Key Points
- Next Chapter Up
- Online/Classroom Discussion
- Learning Activites
  - To-Do List

## REFLECTIVE QUESTIONS

Gaining credible data is a central component of clinical projects. In previous chapters, you considered the importance of developing broad data-collection plans for your project proposal. The following reflective questions help you consider further development of your method section and organize learning for this chapter. As you make a plan for gathering the data, with which of the following are you most confident?

- Why is it important to address detailed plans for data collection?
- What procedures can help make a plan that is systematic and objective?
- What strategies will use to promote confidence in the tools used and the resultant findings?

Use the Practice Scholarship Applications (at the end of this chapter) to help document your learning from concept to competency, including relevant American Association of Colleges of Nursing (AACN) *Essentials* (2021*)*.

When writing a project proposal, addressing the quality of the data to be collected is central. This involves clearly and objectively describing the properties of any data-collection tools and identifying systematic, replicable procedures for data collection. Aligning these components within the project triangle is also key. Building on the varied project plans previously described, this chapter focuses on further detailing the methods component of the project triangle. This also builds on earlier discussions of qualitative and quantitative approaches to interviews, observations, and record reviews. Specific plans for collecting data in systematic, objective, valid, and reliable ways are described in this chapter.

## QUALITY IMPROVEMENT ALERT

The value of your quality improvement (QI) project depends on the quality of your data!

## PROVIDING A DETAILED PLAN FOR DATA COLLECTION

It is helpful to first recall where the proposal-writing process has already taken you and the decisions made. The big picture has included addressing the specific how, when, and what of meaningful data collection. It fits within the purpose, methods, and outcomes points of your project triangle. This chapter further addresses components that need to be detailed within the method section of your clinical project proposal.

## With Your Clinical Project in Mind

What qualitative or quantitative approaches or tools will you be using? How will you describe your tools and your protocols?

- For example, will you be using survey or interview questions that help identify participants' subjective perspectives of knowledge, attitudes, or behaviors?
- Will you be using observations or document review guides to gain data about a specified concept or issue?

Once you decide how data will be collected in your project, you will be naming and clearly describing in your proposal both the tools to be used and the specific protocol or approaches to be followed that can support data accuracy and quality. The following paragraphs further detail how your proposal needs to describe the instruments for data collection and the procedures you will follow. The more complete and thorough the actions you take now with respect to proposed data-collection steps and anticipated problems, the easier the actual implementation of data collection will be later.

## DESCRIBING CREDIBLE/TRUSTWORTHY TOOLS

Recall from Chapter 8 that to evaluate outcomes means to determine how well a project achieved its objectives. You will want to be very specific about the outcomes chosen and how they will be evaluated because, for others to value your work, they need to understand how you have gained the data for your project. You should describe the instruments used and the reliability and validity of these tools (Box 12.1). In describing the data-collection tools/instruments, at minimum, it is necessary to:

- Share a thorough description of the tools, including the number and type of questions. Also include the history of the tool.
- Share any reliability and validity for the tools that have been reported in the literature.

### Share a Thorough Description

As you consider your QI or other DNP project, name the tool you plan to use. Describe briefly the historical development of the tool, including when and how it was developed.

> **BOX 12.1 Describing the Instruments**
>
> **Example 1: Electronic Health Record Survey**
> For a simple survey, the description might begin as follows: This project will use a survey consisting of both closed-ended responses and broad open-ended questions that were developed from items identified in the review of the literature. This descriptive survey includes 12 questions. First, background questions about students' opinions are asked, and then open-ended questions seeking further clarification of students' ideas are posed. This includes 10 structured-response questions (4-point rating) about electronic health records and two open-ended questions. Potential total scores for the 10 structured items range from 10 to 40 (high rating). The full questionnaire is provided in Exhibit 12.1.
>
> **Example 2: Health Behaviors Survey**
> For a more developed survey, the description might begin as follows: A tool developed by Walker et al. (1987), the Health Promoting Lifestyle Profile II, will be used to measure health behaviors. This is a 52-item scale that addresses five subscales of health, including physical activity, nutrition, health responsibility, stress management, and interpersonal relationships. The 52 items are answered using a 4-point response option to indicate subjects' personal habits (*never, sometimes, often,* and *routinely*). The authors reported that high internal consistency reliability and construct validity was confirmed by factor analysis. Further studies have used this tool and also reported >.90 reliability.

Describe examples of other projects that have used this tool. Include strengths and weaknesses of the tool. For example, if you are addressing caring approaches of critical care nurses, your survey could be a tool developed from Watson's work that addressed the 10 carative factors described in Watson's caring theory (Nelson & Watson, 2011). You would note that each of the 10 items is answered using a 4-point scale of 1 (*low*) to 4 (*high*). You would report this description and then provide examples of how other studies have used the tool. This would include further discussion of the tool's qualities, including reliability and validity. In addition, you would note this tool as consistent with the caring theory you chose to guide your study, including consistency with your project definitions of caring. If this is a new tool that was developed from the literature and expert opinion specifically for this project, describe the preceding items as much as possible, including an expert review of the tool.

### Share Reliability and Validity

*Reliability* and *validity* are common research terms. The concept of reliability means methods are dependable or replicable, and the concept of validity means the methods are truthful representations of the data. In describing survey

## EXHIBIT 12.1 SAMPLE SURVEY FORM: OPINIONS ABOUT ELECTRONIC HEALTH RECORDS

**Instructions: Please circle your response to each of the following items.**

1. Learning skills for using an EHR is important in my healthcare profession.

| Strongly disagree | Disagree | Agree | Strongly agree |
|---|---|---|---|

**I plan to use EHRs in the following ways (items 2–6):**

2. Logging patient care

| Strongly disagree | Disagree | Agree | Strongly agree |
|---|---|---|---|

3. Patient progress notes

| Strongly disagree | Disagree | Agree | Strongly agree |
|---|---|---|---|

4. Patient billing purposes

| Strongly disagree | Disagree | Agree | Strongly agree |
|---|---|---|---|

5. Accessing information from other disciplines to support patient care

| Strongly disagree | Disagree | Agree | Strongly agree |
|---|---|---|---|

6. I do not plan to use EHRs in my practice.

| Strongly disagree | Disagree | Agree | Strongly agree |
|---|---|---|---|

**The benefits I see to using EHRs include (items 7–9):**

7. Helping make my documentation more complete

| Strongly disagree | Disagree | Agree | Strongly agree |
|---|---|---|---|

8. Helping minimize errors

| Strongly disagree | Disagree | Agree | Strongly agree |
|---|---|---|---|

9. Helping increase my efficiency

| Strongly disagree | Disagree | Agree | Strongly agree |
|---|---|---|---|

10. I am adequately proficient in EHR skills.

| Strongly disagree | Disagree | Agree | Strongly agree |
|---|---|---|---|

**Instructions: Please write a response to the following items:**

11. The challenges or problems I see to using EHRs include _____
12. Where/when did you receive the most information about using EHRs in your practice? _____

EHR, electronic health record.

*Source:* Bonnel, D. (2011). *Physical therapist assistant students' attitudes towards electronic health records* [Unpublished senior project]. Washburn University.

---

reliability, a common measure to note is internal consistency reliability, or Cronbach's alpha. This indicates how well or reliably the tool has "worked" in the previous studies. Any concepts of validity described in the literature are also noted (such as construct- or criterion-related validity determined from previous work with the tool).

Generally, when projects use qualitative tools, concepts of reliability and validity are described using alternate terms. For example, the term *trustworthiness* considers the concepts of credibility, dependability, and confirmability of qualitative data. Also, potential for transferability of the project findings is considered (Polit & Beck, 2020).

## Describe Related Credibility Issues

Remember that decision trails, which you initiated at the beginning of your project to track decisions, are key tools for establishing and assessing credibility. As you recall, decision trails serve as objective progress records that document processes and decisions from project beginning to end. This is sometimes called an *audit trail* because someone could audit your project decisions or the pathways chosen.

The concept of *triangulation* also has relevance to a credible project. Related to a specific phenomenon, triangulation involves gaining two or more kinds of data; for example, gaining both interview and observation data. An example would be asking children questions about healthy meal choices as well as observing their food choices at a school cafeteria. Using more than one method to obtain a similar result improves the strength of the data (Leedy & Ormrod, 2019).

## Describe the Protocol Procedure for Data Collection

After naming and describing the data-collection tools, you need to indicate a specific procedure for how the tools will be implemented in your project. This section of your proposal involves trustworthy implementation of the protocol for data collection. It is almost a "cookbook"-type approach that someone could replicate. The protocol procedure addresses the administrative what, how, and when questions. For example, if your project involves a patient room-safety observations checklist, you would have already noted your plan to use a tool with good reliability and validity (or gained content-expert review of a checklist you developed from review of the literature). Additional plans to be described in the proposal include approaches such as the following: *Specified observation data from the "safety checklist" will be gained from 10 occupied rooms each weekend over a period of 3 weeks. The safety checklist will be completed by the project director.* As much as can be noted, the protocol procedure further defines the observations, including the who, what, and when of the observations. Another investigator might, for example, want to complete a project that included observations over weekdays to see whether similarities or differences existed.

Similar protocols are needed to plan for interviews or when handing out written surveys. Protocols need to provide enough direction that others could critique a protocol's strengths and weaknesses or replicate the protocol in a similar setting.

### Pilot Test of Tools and Procedures

As you make plans for consistent, reliable data collection, pretesting, or pilot testing, your tools and procedures can help identify any potential problems. Before you hand your survey to 50 potential participants, you want to make sure the setting, procedures, and the survey itself will make them comfortable in responding.

It is important to pilot test your survey form or interview guide since you want to make sure project participants understand the questions you are asking and how to respond honestly. For example, if you are using a qualitative survey and ask, "Could you share an experience about a safety issue?" some respondents might respond yes and then move on. This phrasing, if not caught in a pilot test, would make you miss the opportunity to gather the rich data you were seeking. Piloting would remind you to rephrase this, changing the instruction to something like, "Please share an experience involving a safety issue." Another consideration to keep in mind: If you ask about certain benefits to an item, such as a new staffing plan, and all respondents answer "none," you are also missing data. It is often useful to add a survey question like, "What else would you like to say about this topic?" or "What other thoughts do you have on this topic?"

How many people should you include in the pilot? Although no ideal numbers are noted, at least three people would give you a small range of experiences to get diverse feedback and perspectives. In addition to pilot testing surveys, you should also pilot test observation checklists or document review forms so that others who might use these can help clarify any fuzzy points prior to data collection (Leedy & Ormrod, 2019). Quick tips for planning data collection are noted in Box 12.2.

---

**BOX 12.2 Quick Tips for Data Collection**

You should use good tools and be systematic in using them. Points to consider:

- Describe instruments and procedures (qualitative, quantitative, or mixed) that will be used to gain data or assess the effectiveness of an implementation.
- Report efforts to validate and test reliability of assessment instruments.
- Describe the procedure for collecting the data.
- Include any needed methods for training others in data collection and pilot testing the data-collection plan.

---

## OTHER CONSIDERATIONS

Potential challenges exist in data collection. Address each of the following as part of your method section to promote an efficient and effective project (Krathwohl & Smith, 2005).

### The Setting

Name your setting for data collection. If you plan to have nursing staff complete surveys electronically as part of a face-to-face class, you have to ensure that on a particular day, time, and place, staff will bring or have access to their electronic devices for data entry. An additional consideration in describing the setting or context even includes noting whether you plan to bring snacks for all nursing staff to the classroom. Further evaluating sites for access and appropriateness of the project and data collection are described as part of project feasibility in Chapter 10.

### Data Organization

As data are collected, you will need plans that include logging the data gained. For example, if 50 surveys, all having 20 questions, are completed via paper and pencil, the stack of 50 surveys will not be useful to you. If you are not using an electronic-survey format, your proposal should indicate who will transcribe the data (both numeric and written) and what type of timeline will be used for the transcription. In many cases, this will include first transcribing the data to a program, such as Excel, so that you can review data for completeness and any patterns in responses. Then, in some cases, you will need to transfer the data to a software program for further quantitative or qualitative analyses.

### Storing Data

It is important to address where you will store all collected data. It is especially important to note plans to store your data in a secure place, typically, a locked file that others cannot access. This is required to help you ensure confidentiality of the data. Further issues in ensuring data confidentiality are addressed in Chapter 14.

### Data-Collection Timeline

Your proposal needs a timeline that will guide and promote consistency in data collection and progress (Krathwohl & Smith, 2005). This timeline includes attention to the who, what, and when of data collection. For example, if you are seeking to survey graduating nurses on their readiness to practice in a culture of safety, your survey would likely need to be administered while they were still finishing courses. An error in timelines (or not planning far enough ahead for human subjects or the institutional review board) could make you miss the data-collection point or postpone it by a full semester or even a year. Have a specific timeline in mind of the best time to collect your data.

## Technology and Data Collection

There are both benefits and challenges in using technology in data collection. Benefits include rapid access to surveys for participants and easy access to collected data for the project director. Challenges include ensuring that all participants have easy access to the technologies needed (at the right time and place). In addition, you need reasonable access to online resources that allow you to create or move paper surveys online (Leedy & Ormrod, 2019).

Additional considerations for technology include recognizing its value in gaining secondary data from databases already in existence such as EHRs and the National Database of Nursing Quality Indicators. The value of technology is also noted for organizing and analyzing data. This includes tools, such as spreadsheets, used for organizing, coding, and sorting simple qualitative data or for simple descriptive and basic quantitative data calculations.

## FURTHER CHALLENGES

### Instrument Development

In general, it is best to avoid developing your own instrument for a clinical project, especially if a well-developed instrument already exists. Extensive time and work are involved in instrument development, including recommended graduate coursework. If there is need for a simple survey and none exist in your project area of interest, generating questions supported in the literature or from experience can be a starting point. There are then benefits in gaining review by expert raters, a type of content validity, to support that the questions be asked accurately to reflect the topic you are trying to learn more about.

### Project Internal Validity

Recall from previous coursework that internal validity, or ensuring that the project results are due to your intervention, is critical in making the case for your project findings. You have to help ensure that alternate explanations are not the cause of your outcomes. Controlling variables helps to keep the project as tight as possible to increase confidence in your findings. At minimum, be prepared to discuss variables that may influence your findings. Further reading and consultation with your mentor are needed to address this concept.

It is beneficial to learn from the experience of DNP students who have preceded you in completing project proposals; see Advice From DNP Students.

---

### ADVICE FROM DNP STUDENTS

**Data-Collection Strategies**

Be clear in describing data-collection plans.

- It's not "I will collect data," but instead a detailed description of each point: the who will, when will, and where will data be collected.

Keep your study analysis in mind.

- I am learning more about types of data (nominal, ordinal, interval, and ratio) and that is important because you can only use them in a certain way. That makes a lot of difference in how you choose or set up a tool to gather the information and what you can do with it.

---

### PRACTICE SCHOLARSHIP APPLICATIONS

Consider your competency documentation plans. How will your project address select *Essentials*? Consider additions to your project notebook as you complete the following.

- *Concepts to competence*: Think about your knowledge of collecting credible data. What tools do you plan to use in your project and how do they fit the concepts to be studied? Think about and justify the step-by-step procedures you'll use to collect data.
- *Essentials*: Review the advanced level competencies and subcompetencies for the Knowledge for Nursing Practice and Scholarship for the Nursing Discipline *Essential* domains. Reflect on how they relate to your gaining credible data.
- *Project notebook*: Include a one-page written reflection that addresses the tools you plan to use in your clinical project and why they are considered credible. Self-assess your progress with this chapter as you begin your work.

---

## SUMMARY AND KEY POINTS

This chapter addressed strategies for your clinical project proposal that promote confidence in the tools used and help to ensure that the resultant findings are reliable and valid. Being clear in describing project tools and protocols is key. Points to recall from this chapter include the following:

- Consider strategies for data collection that promote confidence in the data collection plan.
- Describe the features of the tools you are using; in addition, clearly and thoroughly describe the procedures and protocols used for data collection.
- Be systematic and objective as you collect data.
- Remember that decision trails are very important for both establishing and assessing credibility.

- Describe potential credibility issues, such as reliability and validity of the tools used, and consider and report information related to new instrument development.
- Remember to include reports of pilot testing of data-collection tools and QI methods.
- Make sure you have thoroughly described context factors, including the setting and population/sample.

## NEXT CHAPTER UP

After collecting data, you move to analyzing and reporting your data. Strategies for analyzing qualitative data and quantitative data are shared. An important focus will be on extending your descriptive data report to include analysis.

### ONLINE/CLASSROOM DISCUSSION

In discussions with your colleagues, share responses to the following:

- What does it mean to be a clinical scholar? What does your answer have to do with collecting credible data?
- How does collecting credible data add value to your healthcare organization?

## LEARNING ACTIVITIES

### To-Do List

1. Summarize your plan for data collection, including any tools you plan to use and your procedure for data collection, using a one- to two-page abstract-type format.
2. Discuss the strengths and weaknesses of your plan with your mentor. This synthesis of your ideas provides an easy communication tool for your team members.

## REFERENCES

Krathwohl, D., & Smith, N. (2005). *How to prepare a dissertation proposal: Suggestions for students in education and the social and behavioral sciences.* Syracuse University Press.

Leedy, P., & Ormrod, J. (2019). *Practical research: Planning and design* (12th ed.). Pearson.

Nelson, J., & Watson, J. (2011). *Measuring caring: International research on Caritas as healing.* Springer Publishing Company.

Polit, D., & Beck, C. T. (2020). *Nursing research generating and assessing evidence for nursing practice* (11th ed.). Lippincott Williams & Wilkins.

Walker, S., Sechrist, K., & Pender, N. (1987). The health-promoting lifestyle profile: Development and psychometric characteristics. *Nursing Research, 36*(2), 76–81. https://doi.org/10.1097/00006199-198703000-00002

# SECTION III

## Writing Your Proposal: Adding the Detail for Proposal Completion

# 13. Writing the Data-Analysis Plans for Advanced Clinical Projects

## INITIAL THOUGHT

"Data are more than just a list of numbers. They really involve looking for patterns."

## CHAPTER CONTENT

- Reflective Questions
- Quality Improvement Alert
- Plans for Organizing Data
- Plans for Analyzing Data
- The Project Triangle and Data Analysis
- Visualization: Now Consider How You Will Communicate the Data Analysis to Others
- Data-Analysis Considerations
  - Your Proposal: Plan for Descriptive Data and Sample Characteristics
  - Your Proposal: Plan for Sharing Qualitative Results
  - Your Proposal: Plan for Sharing Descriptive Quantitative Results
  - Your Proposal: Plan for Sharing Inferential Quantitative Data-Analysis Results
- Making a Plan for Reporting the Data-Analysis Results: Visual Presentation
- Quick Tips
- Planning Ahead for Project Completion: Discussion/Implications
- Advice From DNP Students
- Practice Scholarship Applications
- Summary and Key Points
- Next Chapter Up
- Online/Classroom Discussions
- Learning Activities
  - To-Do List

## REFLECTIVE QUESTIONS

In Chapter 12, you considered various issues related to collecting valid and reliable data for your proposal plans. In this chapter, you will consider how best to propose plans for analyzing your data. The following reflective questions organize learning for this chapter. With which of the following are you most confident?

- How to organize, analyze, and report the data?
- What strategies and rationales to use for various data-analysis approaches?
- How to write the analysis plan, including addressing benefits/challenges of organizing the full analysis plan in the proposal?

Use the Practice Scholarship Applications (at the end of this chapter) to help document your learning from concept to competency, including relevant American Association of Colleges of Nursing (AACN) *Essentials* (2021).

This chapter focuses on your proposal plans for organizing and analyzing the data you collect for final reporting. Strategies for analyzing subject characteristics, qualitative data, and quantitative data are shared. An important consideration is

### QUALITY IMPROVEMENT ALERT

While data-analysis approaches are described broadly for clinical projects, they also apply to outcome measures in quality improvement (QI) projects. So, this chapter provides a broad discussion of tools that can work well in analyzing QI outcome measures.

on writing plans that focus on analyzing, rather than merely listing, the data obtained. As you write your proposal, this chapter also guides you in thinking it through and anticipating what your final report might look like.

## PLANS FOR ORGANIZING DATA

Advanced clinical projects will include data, whether those data are newly generated data, synthesized from existing data, or evaluation data related to a quality-improvement project. Plans for organizing, analyzing, and reporting those data are important in the proposal plan. Organizing the data essentially involves conveying or listing the data that were collected. The analysis involves a detailed examination that helps you and others better understand or make sense of the data. Too often the plan for data analysis is left out or is just a mere suggestion in a proposal. Reporting data involves communicating the analysis. This plan is needed at the initial proposal stage or you are likely to end up with problems or a gap in what you want to convey.

When planning for organizing, analyzing, and reporting on the data in your proposal, remember that this plan is not an afterthought, but a key component of the project purpose (refer back to the methods point on the project triangle). To accomplish this, the project plan needs to indicate how the collected data will initially be retrieved and organized. This prospective approach also helps ensure that needed data are being collected before it is time for the analysis.

For example, if your project involves surveying 30 people, each responding to 10 survey items, you will want to know their individual responses to items as well as the group's collective responses to items. This allows you to look for patterns, both in individual responses across items as well as the full group response across items. An easy way to gain this big picture of the data is to review the data in an Excel spreadsheet. Creating a "person-by-item" table allows both review of each individual's responses to survey items, seeking any patterns, as well as an opportunity to review summative average responses to each item. Paying "prospective" attention to data analysis is the focus of this chapter.

## PLANS FOR ANALYZING DATA

Although organizing data is an important first step, it is essentially just a listing of the data gathered. Without showing how the data have been reviewed/considered through meaningful analysis, the numbers just become a long laundry list—long lists of data are not very useful unless they are organized into meaningful categories for comparisons. The analysis involves "meaning-making" of the data. For example, you may report the following total scores on a knowledge posttest given to community members about smoking cessation: 75, 34, 89, 52, and 61. However, those scores are meaningless unless accompanied by analysis criteria and interpretation. So, what might have looked like a good, high score of 89 suddenly looks dismal when analysis guidelines indicate a total of 150 points is the possible high score and the higher the score the better.

## THE PROJECT TRIANGLE AND DATA ANALYSIS

Literally, every project will require some type of data analysis. Once your purpose statement, methods, and outcome plans are identified, your detailed method section then provides direction for your analysis plans. The goal is to organize and plan an analysis that ties to the purpose and project questions asked. Thinking through your project analysis requires anticipating what your final report might look like.

Multiple options for completing data analysis exist. For example, most projects will have descriptive statistics that describe sample characteristics. Depending on the project purpose/question and methods, further data gained from this sample may then be presented as descriptive analysis or inferential analysis. Understanding the background of these approaches and why they are important is key. The characteristics of your sample and both qualitative and quantitative analysis approaches are further described in the following sections.

## VISUALIZATION: NOW CONSIDER HOW YOU WILL COMMUNICATE THE DATA ANALYSIS TO OTHERS

Sometimes all the numbers involved in data analysis and presenting its results can be confusing. In this case, it is very helpful to use visuals to make the numbers and findings more easily accessible to others. So communicate appropriate evaluation findings visually when possible. Keep the following points in mind:

- Now, as you're writing your project proposal, is the time to think about and create your visual templates.
- Visuals help to present numeric data using a variety of different formats (e.g., bar graphs, histograms, line graphs, run charts)
- Consider the visual template options and choose the one that best presents each finding; you'll likely use different formats for different findings.
- Initially the visual helps you see what is happening; in addition to making the data clear, the visual draws attention to important results.
- Visuals can then be used in your final report to help the reader clearly see what is happening.
- Make visuals as self-explanatory as possible. If it is a complicated visual, give readers instruction on how to view.
- In your report, complete visuals first and then write the narrative to explain them.
- Use clear titles for visuals that easily convey the content presented.
- Tables and figures should be numbered consecutively throughout your report.
- Additional content and resources about visuals are found at www.ihi.org/insights/5-tips-guiding-improvement-visual-data and www.ihi.org/resources/tools/quality-improvement-essentials-toolkit.

## DATA-ANALYSIS CONSIDERATIONS

### Your Proposal: Plan for Descriptive Data and Sample Characteristics

Your proposal analysis plan will include an initial report of descriptive data. In almost all cases, this will include a descriptive report of the data collected, whether the data are from interviews, surveys, observations, or records reviewed. This means you will have to think ahead about how descriptive data will be shared.

If you are interviewing clinicians, the characteristics you use to describe them will have to match any demographic survey questions you ask them (so you will make sure you have the correct questions on your survey to match what you want to say about the sample). For example, when surveying clinicians, what characteristics about them are important to your clinical project? You likely want to know how many participated and what they "looked" like (e.g., How old are they? How long have they practiced? What are their specialties?).

While you are considering the characteristics you want to describe, it also makes sense to think ahead about how you will report this information. Think ahead about the tables you will want to share after the data are collected. Proposal completion involves detailing even to the point of building blank tables for description, including charts and boxes that hold a place for descriptive findings in your final report.

### Your Proposal: Plan for Sharing Qualitative Results

If you have used a qualitative data-collection approach, such as a survey asking open-ended questions about your topic, you will have to make plans for qualitative data analysis. Your analysis plans will include a review of responses to these open-ended questions to determine common themes. Themes provide a way of conveying what has been learned from long lists of word responses. They offer a way to interpret and make data meaningful. In essence, the goal is to learn how a topic is perceived by subjects or written about in documents (Berg, 2008).

The simple content analysis focuses on themes, messages, or key points in the data. It asks questions about the data that relate back to the study purpose. In some ways, the analysis works as a funnel, first seeking broad pictures from the data and then seeking more specific patterns. The content analysis begins with the following:

- *Review the raw data*: List and consider what has been shared.
- *Organize*: Create files of the data.
- *Examine/peruse*: Prepare an overview, listing preliminary thoughts about the data.
- *Classify*: Put data into categories or themes.
- *Synthesize*: Generate tables or diagrams that outline key themes and, in some cases, hypothesize relationships among the themes.

A *theme* is a simple phrase that captures an idea or concept. Some projects will use a priori coding to seek themes. This means that selected categories are named before the data are reviewed. The categories are then used during the review to see whether they are found in the data. For example, you ask whether the data responses obtained correspond to a set of criteria, such as staff being supportive or unsupportive of a new practice policy. Another approach uses "open" coding. With open coding, themes emerge as common responses when the same responses are heard multiple times. For example, in a qualitative survey of new charge nurses, data might reflect common concerns, or themes, about learning how to staff a unit or engage the team. Themes sometimes emerge when you ask yourself what about the results surprise you.

For example, referring to the sample electronic health record (EHR) survey presented in the previous chapter (see Exhibit 12.1), simple content analysis was used to analyze open-ended question responses (the last two survey items). In completing content analysis of one specific open-ended survey question, "The challenges or problems I see to using EHRs include…," the following themes were identified from the 22 phrases received: issues for training, problems with access, concerns about losing data, and privacy issues. Each theme would then be further described and specific examples for each category provided.

### Your Proposal: Plan for Sharing Descriptive Quantitative Results

Quantitative data analysis provides a way of summarizing your data through numbers. If quantitative data will be gathered, planning choices for analysis include considering whether descriptive statistics only will be appropriate, or will descriptive statistics plus inferential statistics best convey the data findings? In any of the analyses chosen, the goal is to address the project purpose. For example, in planning to evaluate staff satisfaction with a specific staff development program, all responses to a specific survey item (rating 1–4 high) could be summarized according to range, mean, and standard deviation. In addition, the item scores could be averaged for a specific group and their scores reported in a similar fashion. If there is intent to compare satisfaction ratings between new staff and experienced staff, then an inferential statistic, such as the *t*-test, would be used to compare these two groups' mean satisfaction score (a type of inferential statistic). The analysis plan will relate back to the project triangle, with a focus on the methods, including sampling plan and type of data collected (as further described in the following text).

### EXHIBIT 13.1 SAMPLE FREQUENCY COUNT: ELECTRONIC HEALTH RECORD SURVEY

| Items | SD | D | A | SA | Count Total |
|---|---|---|---|---|---|
| 1. | 1 | 0 | 12 | 9 | 22 |
| 2. | 1 | 0 | 15 | 6 | 22 |
| 3. | 0 | 0 | 13 | 9 | 22 |
| 4. | 1 | 0 | 10 | 11 | 22 |
| 5. | 0 | 1 | 11 | 10 | 22 |
| 6. | 13 | 8 | 1 | 0 | 22 |
| 7. | 0 | 0 | 14 | 8 | 22 |
| 8. | 1 | 0 | 14 | 7 | 22 |
| 9. | 1 | 0 | 11 | 10 | 22 |
| 10. | 13 | 6 | 3 | 0 | 22 |

*Note:* Review the sample survey form, EHR Survey, provided in Box 12.1. This example provides data using that tool. The number of respondents for each item option from the sample survey is $N = 22$. Under each of the response categories, the number of total respondents who answered in that category is provided.

A, agree; D, disagree; SA, strongly agree; SD, strongly disagree.

Descriptive quantitative components are a type of counting used to create a numerical picture of the data. They can include a count of contextual elements and might use, for example, tally sheets or frequency counts. These can be created by hand, but technology makes generating these counts fairly easy. Exhibits 13.1 and 13.2 provide examples of tables using frequency counts.

### Your Proposal: Plan for Sharing Inferential Quantitative Data-Analysis Results

If you are using inferential statistics, then you analyze your data to see whether there are unique significant findings (those showing statistical significance) or whether your findings were more probably related to chance. Inferential statistics involve meeting assumptions for inferential statistics (e.g., large sample size, usually noted to be >30 to approximate a normal curve, which the statistics are based on). Data-analysis tests are guided by the level of data being analyzed. To confirm you are choosing the correct inferential tests, you need to describe the level of data in your data collection:

- *Nominal*: This type of data can be put in unique categories in which the answer is one of two options. These include, for example, responses to questions that ask about categories like yes/no or Black/White. For central tendency, modes are reported descriptively, then further analysis with nonparametric tests, such as the chi-square test, can be used for category comparisons.

- *Ordinal*: This type of data can be ordered, such as data from good/better/best-type surveys. These data will typically be reported with medians and ranges; then further analysis can be used with nonparametric tests like the Wilcoxon signed-rank test.

- *Interval/ratio*: This type of data can be used mathematically, such as numerical scores on a knowledge test. Means/averages and standard deviations are reported descriptively, then further analysis is done with parametric statistics, such as *t*-tests, analysis of variance (ANOVA), or other tests, depending on the project purpose.

Once you identify the level of data, return to your handy statistics textbook to confirm you are planning the right test for your type of data (consulting with your mentor is also a good idea). For instance, in a continuing-education program example, it might be appropriate to compare mean program satisfaction scores between new staff and experienced staff using an independent *t*-test.

A good guide for those new to advanced clinical project data-analysis plans is to select only the core variables for simple inferential testing. Again, indicate any plans to complete simple inferential tests as part of the project proposal. As you work on this section of your proposal, you will want additional readings and references to support your plans. If you are new to this process, a useful reference, such as *Statistics for People Who (Think They) Hate Statistics* (Salkind, 2016), can be helpful. More complex approaches to analysis can be considered with your mentor.

## MAKING A PLAN FOR REPORTING THE DATA-ANALYSIS RESULTS: VISUAL PRESENTATION

Even though you have no data at the proposal stage, making plans to organize your descriptive data and data analyses provides a step up when it is time for the analysis phase of your project. Consider the value of using a large three-ring binder or its electronic equivalent. If your final project report will end with the traditional five scholarly sections, put five dividers in this binder at the beginning of project implementation as a reminder of, or placeholder for, the final sections; adjust accordingly for the sections required in your own program format. This basically requires visualizing, at the proposal stage, the project as processed and completed. In preparation for the data you will soon acquire, data-analysis plans can even include the blank table formats. Although this advice is easy to ignore, addressing this advice will pay dividends in saved time and frustration later.

As you plan to communicate your final project results, you will want to visually showcase these in your final project paper. Generate plans for tables or charts that can be used to document descriptive characteristics of project subjects as well as further data analyses from surveys or other tools.

## EXHIBIT 13.2 PERSON-BY-ITEM DESCRIPTIVE RESULTS: ELECTRONIC HEALTH RECORD SURVEY

| Items | 1 | 2 | 3 | 4 | 5 | 6 | 7 | 8 | 9 | 10 |
|---|---|---|---|---|---|---|---|---|---|---|
| Subject 1 | 3 | 3 | 3 | 2 | 3 | 2 | 3 | 3 | 2 | 2 |
| 2 | 3 | 3 | 3 | 4 | 1 | 3 | 3 | 3 | 3 | 2 |
| 3 | 3 | 3 | 3 | 3 | 3 | 1 | 4 | 4 | 4 | 1 |
| 4 | 3 | 3 | 3 | 3 | 3 | 1 | 3 | 3 | 3 | 2 |
| 5 | 3 | 3 | 3 | 3 | 3 | 2 | 3 | 3 | 3 | 1 |
| 6 | 4 | 4 | 4 | 4 | 4 | 2 | 3 | 3 | 3 | 2 |
| 7 | 4 | 4 | 3 | 3 | 4 | 2 | 3 | 3 | 4 | 2 |
| 8 | 3 | 3 | 3 | 3 | 3 | 2 | 3 | 3 | 3 | 2 |
| 9 | 4 | 3 | 4 | 4 | 3 | 2 | 4 | 4 | 4 | 2 |
| 10 | 4 | 3 | 3 | 3 | 4 | 2 | 3 | 3 | 3 | 3 |
| 11 | 3 | 3 | 3 | 3 | 3 | 2 | 3 | 3 | 3 | 1 |
| 12 | 4 | 4 | 4 | 4 | 4 | 1 | 4 | 4 | 4 | 2 |
| 13 | 3 | 3 | 3 | 3 | 3 | 2 | 3 | 3 | 3 | 1 |
| 14 | 4 | 3 | 4 | 4 | 4 | 1 | 4 | 4 | 4 | 2 |
| 15 | 2 | 3 | 3 | 3 | 4 | 2 | 3 | 2 | 4 | 1 |
| 16 | 4 | 3 | 3 | 4 | 3 | 2 | 3 | 4 | 4 | 2 |
| 17 | 3 | 4 | 4 | 4 | 4 | 1 | 4 | 3 | 4 | 3 |
| 18 | 3 | 3 | 3 | 3 | 3 | 1 | 3 | 3 | 3 | 2 |
| 19 | 3 | 4 | 4 | 4 | 4 | 1 | 4 | 3 | 3 | 3 |
| 20 | 3 | 3 | 4 | 4 | 3 | 2 | 3 | 4 | 4 | 2 |
| 21 | 4 | 4 | 4 | 4 | 4 | 1 | 4 | 4 | 4 | 2 |
| 22 | 3 | 3 | 4 | 4 | 4 | 2 | 3 | 3 | 3 | 1 |
| **Average** | 3.30 | 3.27 | 3.41 | 3.45 | 3.36 | 1.68 | 3.31 | 3.27 | 3.41 | 1.86 |
| **Standard Deviation** | 0.57 | 0.46 | 0.50 | 0.60 | 0.73 | 0.57 | 0.48 | 0.55 | 0.59 | 0.64 |
| **Mode** | 3 | 3 | 3 | 4 | 3 | 2 | 3 | 3 | 3 | 2 |
| **Median** | 3 | 3 | 3 | 3.5 | 3 | 2 | 3 | 3 | 3 | 2 |

*Note*: Again, review the EHR survey form provided in Box 12.1. This table provides basic descriptive data showing how each of the 22 respondents marked each survey item. Setting up a table such as this allows you to look for patterns.

Tables and charts help organize data that are too complex to just convey through paragraph form. Those who read your final project paper will often find it easiest to skim your tables and charts to quickly identify findings. Creating these placeholders now, for future data, also provides you an opportunity to confirm you are collecting the correct data to address your purpose statement. Making this plan now may even make it easier to complete the write-up of these sections as you work with these established tables (Box 13.1).

## QUICK TIPS

Sometimes it is easiest to start by sharing the descriptive data and then summarizing how these data answer the project question(s). At minimum include the following:

- *Subject demographics*: Descriptive statistics are used to share demographic data. Share your plans for completing tables or bullets with frequencies and ranges of responses for each demographic item.

> **BOX 13.1 Writing the Data-Analysis Plan**
>
> The following paragraph provides a sample analysis plan for a hypothetical EHR project. The project's purpose is to identify perceptions of graduating students on readiness to use EHRs in their employment settings after graduation. Using the EHR survey example supplied in Box 12.1, the following paragraph provides a brief summary evaluation plan for the 10-item quantitative survey and two-item qualitative questions.
>
> *Data analysis will be completed with basic descriptive statistics used to describe responses to the 10 structured-response items. An Excel spreadsheet of each participant's responses will be shared (Exhibits 13.1 and 13.2). This allows review of the numeric data for patterns. A frequency-count table will be constructed to further analyze subject responses with appropriate histograms generated. Qualitative responses to the two open-ended items will be typed verbatim into a word-processing program. Content analysis seeking themes will be completed by the researcher and a second health professional.*

- *Closed-ended (limited response) items*: Descriptive statistics are used to convey responses to survey items that are close ended. Share plans for completing tables or bullets with frequencies and central tendency measures for each item on a survey or checklist (as well as total scores if using a validated tool).
- *Open-ended (descriptive response) items*: Simple content analysis leads to descriptive themes from open-ended survey items. Plan to share common themes identified from these items; for example, in bullet-list form or a summary table.

## PLANNING AHEAD FOR PROJECT COMPLETION: DISCUSSION/IMPLICATIONS

After implementing your proposal and completing your project data analysis, you will establish conclusions and recommendations. These are based on the synthesis of evidence from your project and related to your project purpose. These sections will help you address the "so what" of findings from the project.

Even in the planning phase, it is important to consider potential project implications. Often, implications will be considered, at minimum, in terms of further implications for practice, education, and research. For example, in the EHR project example in this chapter, the following implications might emerge for the discussion section of a final report:

- *Implication for practice*: It is important for academic and practice settings to work together in preparing students for future clinical work with EHRs.
- *Implications for education*: Further education is recommended across classroom and clinical settings.
- *Implications for further research*: Further study of the best ways to learn and use EHRs is recommended.

> **ADVICE FROM DNP STUDENTS**
>
> **Data-Analysis Strategies**
>
> Know analysis plans prior to collecting data.
>
> - I learned that it is imperative to think about and have an idea of the type of data you will obtain, how you will utilize it, and why you chose the method of analysis you did.
> - Know ahead of time what statistics you will use. This serves as a check and helps make sure you are gaining the right data.
>
> Know levels of data.
>
> - Walk away understanding nominal, ordinal, interval, and ratio data. I never understood the terms before.
>
> Think about tools available to you.
>
> - Learn about programs, like Excel, that you can use to manage data.
>
> Appreciate the value of showing or providing visuals of the data.
>
> - Create blank tables as part of the proposal. Become savvy in use of tables and graphs for data visualization.
>
> Don't write about an analysis that will not apply.
>
> - The most challenging parts for me are trying to determine the data analysis that will be utilized for my project and creating tables before you even have the data.
>
> Use your previous coursework on research and epidemiology.
>
> - Pull out the practical/applied stats book and review statistics that you will need for your project.

> **PRACTICE SCHOLARSHIP APPLICATIONS**
>
> Consider your competency documentation plans. How will your project address select *Essentials*? Consider additions to your project notebook as you complete the following.
>
> - *Concepts to competence*: Think about your knowledge about reporting data-analysis results. What analysis procedures will you use and why? How will you visually display your analysis results?
> - *Essentials*: Review the advanced-level competencies and subcompetencies for the Knowledge for Nursing Practice and Scholarship for the Nursing Discipline *Essential* domains. Reflect on how they relate to your data analysis.
> - *Project notebook*: Include a one-page written reflection that addresses (a) your specific data-analysis plan and (b) the templates of how you'll help others visualize your analysis findings.

After project implementation, your results and discussion/implications sections will be components of your final project report. Plan to create a scholarly document to be presented and defended to your community of interest as well as other stakeholders, academic communities, and interested parties.

As you move forward in your work, consider the experiences of DNP students who have already completed project proposals. Their advice is presented in the Advice From DNP Students box.

## SUMMARY AND KEY POINTS

Planning for data collection and analysis in your project go hand in hand. Proactive planning helps avoid the problem of gaining too much, not enough, or the wrong data. This chapter provided direction for thinking ahead to final components of the project, including organizing and analyzing the data you collect. You will want to make credible plans for data analysis so that all can clearly understand your project results. Points to recall from this chapter include the following:

- Provide a detailed plan for data review, organization, and analysis. Be systematic and objective.
- Clearly and thoroughly describe your plan for data analysis so that all can clearly understand how you obtained your project results.
- Remember to describe a specific plan for sharing broad descriptive data collected, including sample characteristics.
- If you are sharing qualitative data-analysis results, your proposal plan will likely call for simple content analysis or seeking themes from the data.
- If you are sharing descriptive quantitative results, your proposal plan will include describing the inferential statistics to be used and the rationale for using them.
- Think ahead to the visual presentation of the results of data analysis, including completion of templates for graphs and tables.
- Plan ahead for project completion, including discussion of findings and potential project implications.

## NEXT CHAPTER UP

Being ethical and accountable in your project work is a key component of clinical scholarship. Key ethical issues for project proposals are addressed in Chapter 14.

### ONLINE/CLASSROOM DISCUSSION

In discussion with your colleagues, share responses to the following:

- Share a summary page including your purpose statement, triangle points, data-analysis plans, and template for sharing your results.
- Serving as a peer reviewer, provide feedback that includes both strengths and weaknesses of each classmate's data-analysis plans and visual templates for presenting the results.

## LEARNING ACTIVITIES

### To-Do List

Review your data-analysis plans and address the following questions:

1. What is your level of data?
2. What are your analysis plans?
3. How do your plans flow from your project purpose statement?
4. How does your proposal set the stage for displaying and discussing your results?
5. Does your mentor agree with your analysis plans?

## REFERENCES

Berg, B. (2008). *Qualitative research methods for the social sciences* (7th ed.). Pearson.

Salkind, N. (2016). *Statistics for people who (think they) hate statistics* (6th ed.). Sage.

# 14. Keeping Clinical Projects Ethical and Dependable

## INITIAL THOUGHT

"What is the right way to do the right thing?"

## CHAPTER CONTENT

- Reflective Questions
- Quality Improvement Alert
- Professionalism and Professional Standards
- Key Ethical Issues
  - Give Credit Where Credit Is Due: Avoiding Plagiarism
  - Permission to Use Instruments
  - Conflict of Interest
  - Human Subjects and Institutional Review Boards
  - Diversity and Inclusion
  - Data Integrity and Use
  - Artificial Intelligence
- Final Steps
- Summary and Key Points
- Practice Scholarship Applications
- Websites for Further Review
- Next Chapter Up
- Online/Classroom Discussion
- Learning Activities
  - To-Do List

## REFLECTIVE QUESTIONS

You have spent a lot of time working on your project. You have identified concepts of interest, reviewed and organized the literature, honed the purpose statement, and determined what methods and data analysis you will use. One issue that impacts all of these activities is how to do all of this in an ethical manner. The following reflective questions organize learning for this chapter. With which of the following are you most confident?

- How do professional competencies and standards extend to clinical projects?
- Why are ethical issues important in clinical projects?
- What do these concepts mean in planning and writing a project proposal?

Use the Practice Scholarship Applications (at the end of this chapter) to help document your learning from concept to competency, including relevant American Association of Colleges of Nursing (AACN) *Essentials* (2021).

## QUALITY IMPROVEMENT ALERT

Ethical principles are key in all nursing activities, so consider the following chapter content as it applies to your quality improvement (QI) project as well!

## PROFESSIONALISM AND PROFESSIONAL STANDARDS

Since you read about plans for analyzing your data in the last chapter, you may feel like you are about done with your clinical project proposal. However, some of the most important content has been saved for last. Your project will not receive the desired recognition or acceptance if it has not been conducted with the utmost integrity, and so you need to be sure that all ethical aspects of the project have been identified and addressed.

All nurses must adhere to nursing's professional values and standards. Standards have been established by a number of professional nursing organizations to guide the implementation of those values. The American Nurses Association's *Scope and Standards of Practice* (2022) and *Code of Ethics for Nurses With Interpretive Statements* (2015) are two such documents. When you move into scholarly work with your clinical project, additional standards and competencies apply. For example, when writing a formal paper, such as a proposal, a specific writing style is identified and applied. In nursing, that is often the format suggested by the American Psychological Association (APA, 2020), although other styles may also be used. Note that periodically the APA manual is updated with a new edition, and that is a good thing. For example, as more and more references are found online, APA expanded the guidelines for documenting such finds. Other changes in the newest, seventh edition, include no longer identifying the place of publication for books on the reference list. A brief summary of additional changes in the seventh edition of the APA (2020) publication manual is available (www.scribbr.com/apa-style/apa-seventh-edition-changes).

Writing with integrity means more than simply following the assigned writing style (although, along with a variety of other standards, the APA guidelines also address many key ethical standards). Ethical standards and competencies extend beyond nursing to interprofessional teamwork. For example, *Core Competencies for Interprofessional Collaborative Practice* (Interprofessional Education Collaborative Expert Panel, 2011) includes competency domains for values and ethics for interprofessional practice, roles and responsibilities, interprofessional communication, and teams and teamwork. Also, whenever you participate in conducting research on human subjects, the Federal Policy for the Protection of Human Subjects (2018) details pertinent guidelines. Using these documents can be key to completing successful professional projects with the required professional integrity.

## KEY ETHICAL ISSUES

In early nursing profession curricula, you learned about ethical principles such as respect, beneficence, nonmaleficence, autonomy, justice, veracity, and fidelity. These ethical principles, which include doing good, respecting independence, being fair, and being truthful, apply just as much to your clinical project as they do to providing patient care. Oftentimes multiple ethical principles may be involved in the same situation. Some important aspects of applying ethical principles in your clinical project follow.

### Give Credit Where Credit Is Due: Avoiding Plagiarism

Recognizing and acknowledging the work of others is a fundamental element of scholarly writing, as you need to truthfully acknowledge who originated those thoughts and words (veracity). So whenever you use someone else's exact words, or even someone else's ideas paraphrased in your own words, you must give that person credit. Failure to recognize ideas and words that belong to someone else as their work, and not yours, constitutes plagiarism. Although this may seem like a simple concept, it can be deceptive. There is no problem when you are the author of a paper (the clinical project proposal, or any paper on which you are acknowledged as the author) and you include ideas that are your own thoughts that are written in your own words, and that you have never published before. You can simply write them down and move on.

A deceptive and slightly more complicated case is when you are writing about your own thoughts, but you have previously published these thoughts. In this case, and because of copyright laws, you must reference your previous thoughts, even though they all came from you. The failure to reference your own previous work is called *self-plagiarism*.

A much clearer example of plagiarism is when you use or refer to someone else's ideas or words and fail to give that person credit. Credit is given by correctly referencing the source of the words or ideas, so that readers can go to that source and see the original words or ideas themselves. The practice of referencing has very important implications for your proposal.

- When you use someone else's exact words, you must insert quotation marks or italicize their words and provide the source in which those exact words can be found.
- When you use someone else's ideas, even if you paraphrase the ideas using your own words to describe the other person's ideas, then you must also provide the source in which that exact idea can be found.
- Whether you paraphrase someone else's ideas or place quotation marks around their exact words, any citation you reference in the text of your paper must also be placed in the reference list at the end of your document.
- Provide the source in which those words and/or ideas that you are referencing can be found exactly as prescribed by the writing style you are using.

### Permission to Use Instruments

Although any number of instruments are available for use in the public domain and may therefore be used by anyone (with appropriate referencing, of course), there are a number of instruments that do not fall into that category. Permission is required to use instruments that are unpublished and developed by someone else, as well as instruments that have been copyrighted. This standard is based on being truthful (veracity) about who developed the instrument and respectful of their copyright, as to not respect their copyright breaches both ethical and legal principles. In both cases, you must receive formal permission to use the instruments, and that written permission must be (a) referenced in the proposal narrative and (b) provided in the appendices.

### Conflict of Interest

Conflict of interest occurs when project leaders do not maintain unbiased objectivity in a project because they have something at stake or have competing interests—most often, but not always, they have something to gain (Steneck, 2007). Justice is one ethical principle involved with conflict of interest, as it is unfair to give oneself an advantage over others. Potential financial gain is frequently the first example of a conflict of interest that can be identified. Conflicts of interest may also include competing responsibilities or benefits of either a personal or professional nature. A clear example of conflict of interest is seen when a company conducts research on its own product and concludes, contrary to objective analysis of the data, that the product is excellent, not harmful, and should be widely used. Another example is when drug representatives conduct a presentation or provide gifts or meals that encourage use of their products over a competitor's, when their competitor has no chance to respond on behalf of their own products. A more subtle example might be a student who participates in a project with a boss, professor, or admired colleague, in which case objectivity might be lost to the advantage of the boss, professor, or colleague. Conflicts, when they exist, do not necessarily mean that the project cannot be completed. Rather, use of a completely honest and transparent process that identifies the conflict(s) and applies mechanisms by which objectivity can be maintained and monitored must be implemented and documented.

## Human Subjects and Institutional Review Boards

The most comprehensive standards in any clinical project are those regarding the use of human subjects (there are also comprehensive standards for projects that include the use of animals, although that is far less common in nursing and so is not addressed in this book). All project leaders conducting research are expected to uphold the ethical principles of autonomy, justice, and beneficence (Steneck, 2007) through the self-regulation of their respective professions. That self-regulation is augmented by federal government legislation, which was formalized in 1974 when the Department of Health, Education and Welfare codified the procedures of research under Title 45 of the Code of Federal Regulations, part 46 (Federal Policy for the Protection of Human Subjects, 2018). In 1991, most federal agencies affiliated with human research adopted common regulation for human subject protections as 45 CFR 46, subpart A, which is commonly referred to as the *Common Rule* (Federal Policy for the Protection of Human Subjects, 2018).

Institutional review boards (IRBs) are established to implement and monitor the principles of research promulgated in the Common Rule at all institutions receiving federal dollars. Although many clinical projects do not constitute research per se, it is the IRB (and not the project leader) who makes that determination. The general rule is that clinical project proposals need to be reviewed (or at least screened) by the IRB. If the clinical project is deemed "exempt," further IRB oversight may not be required. Project decisions and classifications are the IRB's purview and not determined by the investigators themselves. Working with your faculty mentor, you must receive the IRB's decision regarding your project's status before implementing your project.

Each institution has its own specific policies and procedures on how the Common Rule is implemented, and so it is your responsibility to know the policies and procedures for your own institution. For example, in some institutions, students do not interact directly with the IRB; rather, students work with their faculty advisors, and then the faculty interacts with the IRB. In other places, after students have consulted

> **BOX 14.1 Agency Website**
>
> Visit the website(s) of your institution(s) to see what policies and procedures exist with relevance to your project proposal. Keep in mind that if you hold multiple roles (such as student and employee), or if you will use multiple project sites, you must comply with the regulations of all involved institutions.

faculty and completed required forms, students themselves interact directly with the IRB. Keep in mind, too, that if you are associated with multiple institutions and/or will conduct the project at multiple sites, all of those sites/institutions must review the proposal and provide written approval. Be sure you know and follow your organization's procedures (Box 14.1) and remember that no aspect of the project may be started until the proposal has been reviewed and you have received written notification or approval to proceed from the IRB.

If the IRB deems your clinical project as research, you will likely be required to complete training such as the Collaborative Institutional Training Initiative (CITI) before beginning your project. The CITI training website is easily accessible online. The program consists of several modules, which do not need to be completed all at the same time. Depending on your previous knowledge, the basic course of modules usually takes several hours to complete.

If a clinical project is research that involves human subjects, you must address informed consent. Informed consent is one of the most complex features of the Common Rule and is closely monitored by IRBs, as it is a primary mechanism by which the ethical principles of autonomy, justice, and beneficence are upheld when human subjects are involved in projects. Exhibit 14.1 provides direction if your clinical project is determined to be research and a consent form is needed for human subject participation.

The implications of the Common Rule are far-reaching for all students and project directors conducting clinical projects with human subjects. The good news is that you only need to know that virtually all projects need to be screened by the IRB and a written decision regarding the status of each project must be received from the IRB before implementation can begin. Projects involving human subjects and identified as research will require continuing oversight from the IRB. This IRB review process takes time and so you need to account for that in your projected clinical project timeline.

## Diversity and Inclusion

Current research and project guidelines aim to minimize issues of discrimination based on race, gender, age, and other diversity characteristics, as all have to do with the ethical principle of justice. One way this ethical principle is important in clinical projects is in the topics that projects address. Inequities in healthcare (National Academies, 2024),

## EXHIBIT 14.1 PROTECTION OF HUMAN SUBJECTS

If the IRB determines that your clinical project research will involve human subjects, then you must inform potential participants of

- the project's background, purpose, and procedures;
- why they have been asked to participate;
- their right to not participate, without any negative repercussions;
- their right to withdraw from the project at any time without negative repercussions;
- their right to ask questions about participation;
- their right to voluntarily consent to participate without coercion;
- their right to know the benefits of participating, as well as any risks or inconveniences;
- their right to confidentiality; and
- their access to the project leader's contact information in case they have questions or are injured.

With this information, and being as fully informed as possible, potential participants are able to make autonomous decisions about their willingness to participate in a project or not.

In addition to protecting the autonomy of all potential research participants, IRBs work to protect vulnerable populations whose autonomy may be limited. The Common Rule has in place additional protections for certain groups, such as pregnant women, human fetuses, neonates, children, and prisoners, who may be asked to participate in research studies. Many social determinants of health (environmental conditions in which people are born and/or live that affect their health and quality of life), such as exposure to crime and violence, language/literacy, and socioeconomic conditions (U.S. Department of Health and Human Services, n.d.), may also affect potential research participants' ability to exercise full autonomy in choosing to participate in research or not. All project proposals must demonstrate your thorough analysis and plan for protecting all potential participants, especially those who, for whatever reason, may be considered vulnerable in their ability to make autonomous decisions.

Several organizations provide consent-form templates for project directors. Go to your own institution's website and see whether you can find an example. If you do not find a template at your own organization, or if you want to compare templates, an example is provided on the University of Missouri–Kansas City's website (https://ors.umkc.edu/services/compliance/irb/informed-consent.html).

---

considered as diverse characteristics (such as race, ethnicity, age, gender, and socioeconomic status), can impact poor health outcomes. Clinical projects that address these disparities and the social determinants of health that lead to them can provide important contributions to a just society.

In addition to project topics, the ethical principle of justice also impacts both clinical project teams and the selected project participants, as they need to reflect the diverse populations they are intended to represent. Groups, like Black, Indigenous, and people of color (BIPOC) and Black, Asian, and minority ethnic (BAME), help keep visible the need for equal and fair opportunities to conduct and participate in activities such as clinical projects. Health disparities and social determinants of health (U.S. Department of Health and Human Services, n.d.) affect potential human subjects' ability to participate in clinical projects and provide a growing topic for potential clinical projects as well.

Written statements in your proposal that are relevant to fair representation need to be addressed. Additionally, the APA (2020) manual, for example, includes an entire section on bias-free language. Efforts to give all people equal opportunity to participate in clinical projects must be made and documented.

## Data Integrity and Use

You are nearing completion of your project proposal and you already have a wealth of time and effort invested. It is imperative that you take the time now and follow the steps necessary to ensure the dependability (relating to the ethical principles of veracity) of the data you will collect and use because, without that, your reputation and the impact of your hard work will not be respected by the scholarly community and practicing nurses.

You have already anticipated and addressed several threats to dependable and reliable or trustworthy and transferable data during the design and data-collection procedures of your project. For example, you chose reliable instruments and may have used triangulation approaches to gain trustworthy perspectives. Now you must also ensure the integrity of the data through ongoing, accurate, confidential, and dependable record keeping. This process is often facilitated by keeping an ongoing log of your project activities and decisions, as captured in a decision trail.

What you do with the data you have collected is also important. If you have hard copies of data, such as completed surveys, be sure they are stored in a secure and locked location, such as a locked file cabinet. If you have data saved electronically, be sure that the files are protected by a strong password that is not shared with others who do not have permission to access the records. Be sure to check the policies and procedures at your own institution(s) to confirm how long you must keep and maintain your project data and files.

Also, be sure that you follow all regulations regarding the use and sharing of data, such as the Health Insurance Portability and Accountability Act (HIPAA; Centers for Disease Control and Prevention, 1996), which addresses the confidential use of personal health information, including disclosure and access issues. In addition to addressing how patient data can be used, it discusses obligations to protect that information in its use.

## Artificial Intelligence

Artificial intelligence (AI) can be an incredible resource that potentially affects many aspects of the clinical project. In writing your project proposal, AI tools such as Microsoft Editor are well accepted as they help with features such as grammar and spell checks. In other words, some basic elements of AI are already embedded in what are considered acceptable practices.

Beyond that, keep in mind that sets of facts gained from AI may be from unvetted sources and not credible for scholarly papers. AI cannot reason or make decisions (DeGagne, 2023). The writing produced by AI is based on predictions of word order gleaned from the sources they have analyzed. Furthermore, simply entering topic words into an AI program so that AI does the writing for you may be another form of plagiarism. While AI has value in healthcare, its exponential expansion suggests that new ethical issues, which have not been previously considered, will grow rapidly.

## FINAL STEPS

There are lots of ethical aspects to clinical projects and other scholarly work. The best advice is to be well informed on the ethical issues and to address them up front, during the proposal phase of your clinical project. Remember to consult with project mentors on any questions. This is not an area where it is best to "ask for forgiveness afterward," so be proactive and transparent in your preparations. Go through the entire list of ethical aspects, be absolutely honest with yourself and your team, and address each item now.

## SUMMARY AND KEY POINTS

This chapter has presented issues related to conducting your project in an ethical manner. Working through the IRB process can add unexpected time to the project and may result in the addition of safeguards that you had not previously considered, but the additional effort in respecting not only the integrity of your work, but also the integrity of any participants who may be a part of your work, is an essential element of the scholarly process. Points to recall from this chapter include the following:

- Conducting a clinical project means adhering to scholarship and research-focused values and standards.
- Always give credit to other people whose ideas you may incorporate into your own clinical project.
- Obtain permission to use unpublished and copyrighted instruments.

> **PRACTICE SCHOLARSHIP APPLICATIONS**
>
> Consider your competency documentation plans. How will your project address select *Essentials*? Consider additions to your project notebook as you complete the following.
>
> - *Concepts to competence*: As you review this chapter, think about your knowledge of ethical principles and their impact on your clinical project proposal. Review your project proposal and be sure all information from authors other than yourself are properly cited in your narrative and properly listed in your references. If IRB review is indicated, identify the timeline for IRB review of your project proposal.
> - *Essentials*: Review the advanced level competencies and subcompetencies of the Knowledge for Nursing Practice, Scholarship for the Nursing Discipline, and Professionalism domains. Reflect specifically on the competencies of professionalism and consider their application to your own clinical project.
> - *Project notebook*: Include your completed reference list following APA (or your own program's writing guidelines) format. Include your completed IRB application (as required by your institution and program), as well as letter(s) of permission to conduct proposed project.

- Be sure to acknowledge and address potential conflicts of interest you may have in a clinical project.
- If your project includes research activities, follow guidelines in Title 45 of the Code of Federal Regulations (the Common Rule) to protect human subjects participating in your project.
- Be familiar with, and follow, all federal regulations, such as HIPAA.
- Be familiar with and follow your own institution's research policies and procedures.
- Diversity and inclusion are key elements in not only selecting clinical project topics, but also selecting the project team and participants.
- AI can be a wonderful resource, but requires close attention to ethical standards in order to be used appropriately.

## WEBSITES FOR FURTHER REVIEW

Further examples of tools used for ethical decision-making that can be applied when considering clinical projects include the following:

- The Critical Thinking series provides sample documents on ethics and opportunities to gain further tools relevant to your project plans. *The Thinker's Guide to Ethical Reasoning* sample provides further information:

    www.criticalthinking.org/store/products/ethical-reasoning/169

Social determinants have a huge impact on health and related clinical projects. Read more about social determinants of health at the following:

- *A Framework for Educating Health Professionals to Address the Social Determinants of Health*: www.nap.edu/catalog/21923/a-framework-for-educating-health-professionals-to-address-the-social-determinants-of-health

## NEXT CHAPTER UP

You now have a fairly complete proposal in hand, and you have addressed the ethical elements and ramifications of the project as well. Your next step is to edit, revise, and finalize the proposal so that it is ready for others to review. As you revise and edit, you will be laying the groundwork for your final project paper, which will have widespread distribution—even publication—and you want everything to be accurate as well as conducive to finishing that final report.

### ONLINE/CLASSROOM DISCUSSION

In discussions with your colleagues, share responses to the following:

- Remember the basic ethical principles such as respect, beneficence, nonmaleficence, autonomy, justice, veracity, and fidelity. In what ways will each of these need to be addressed in your proposal?

## LEARNING ACTIVITIES

### To-Do List

If your project requires consent forms, use your agency's template to start a draft of your consent form, being sure to include

- the name of the project and project team;
- why any individuals are being asked to participate;
- a brief rationale for the project and participation;
- a brief explanation of the project's purpose;
- a brief explanation of the project procedures and the nature of the participants' activities and time commitment;
- the benefits (including any payment/compensation);
- the risks of participation (including fees);
- that participation is voluntary, with no negative consequences if individuals choose not to participate or choose to withdraw at any time, as well as alternatives to participation;
- confidentiality details;
- who to contact with questions/problems/injury; and
- signature block for participant and consenter.

_____

_____

_____

_____

_____

_____

_____

_____

## REFERENCES

American Nurses Association. (2015). *Code of ethics for nurses with interpretive statements*. https://www.nursingworld.org/practice-policy/nursing-excellence/ethics/code-of-ethics-for-nurses/

American Nurses Association. (2022). *Scope and standards of practice* (4th ed.).

American Psychological Association. (2020). *Publication manual of the American Psychological Association* (7th ed.).

Centers for Disease Control and Prevention. (1996). *Health insurance portability and accountability act*. https://www.cdc.gov/phlp/php/resources/health-insurance-portability-and-accountability-act-of-1996-hipaa.html

DeGagne, J. C. (2023, March 10). The state of artificial intelligence in nursing education: Past, present, and future directions. *International Journal of Environmental Research and Public Health, 20*(6), 4884. https://doi.org/10.3390/ijerph20064884

Federal Policy for the Protection of Human Subjects. (2018). *45 CFR 46.* http://www.hhs.gov/ohrp/humansubjects/guidance/45cfr46.html

Interprofessional Education Collaborative Expert Panel. (2011). *Core competencies for interprofessional collaborative practice: Report of an expert panel*. https://ipec.memberclicks.net/assets/2011-Original.pdf

National Academies. (2024). *Ending unequal treatment: Strategies to achieve equitable health care and optimal health for all*. https://nap.nationalacademies.org/catalog/27820/ending-unequal-treatment-strategies-to-achieve-equitable-health-care-and

Steneck, N. H. (2007). *Office of research integrity: Introduction to the responsible conduct of research*. http://ori.hhs.gov/documents/rcrintro.pdf

U.S. Department of Health and Human Services. (n.d.). Social determinants of health. *Healthy People 2030*. https://odphp.health.gov/healthypeople/priority-areas/social-determinants-health

# 15. Finalizing the Proposal as a Professional Document: Reviewing, Editing, and Revising

## INITIAL THOUGHT

"Be prepared to revise your proposal multiple times!"

## CHAPTER CONTENT

- Reflective Questions
- Quality Improvement Alert
- Revising the First Draft
- Completing the Final Proposal: Questions to Guide Your Writing
  - Proposal Substance
  - Proposal Structure
  - Proposal Appendices
  - Writing and Editing
- Additional Writing Tips
- Finalizing the Timeline and Project Budget
  - What Is the Project Timeline?
  - What Is the Project Budget?
- Tools That Facilitate Proposal Completion
  - The Project Team and Committee
  - Peer Review
  - Self-Review and Your Decision Trail
- Reflecting and Self-Editing
- Presenting Your Proposal From the Podium
- Next Steps: Using the Proposal for Project Implementation and Final Report Write-Up
- Advice From DNP Students
- Practice Scholarship Applications
- Summary and Key Points
- Next Chapter Up
- Online/Classroom Discussions
- Learning Activities
  - Peer Feedback
  - To-Do List

## REFLECTIVE QUESTIONS

In Chapter 14, you reviewed considerations for proposing and conducting your project in an ethical manner. In this chapter, you approach the final step of editing, revising, and finalizing your proposal so that it is ready for others to review. The following reflective questions organize learning for this chapter. With which of the following are you most confident?

- How to finalize the proposal draft (including edits/revisions) as a professional document?
- What are the next steps in using the proposal to move toward project completion?
- How to use of self-assessment and the project team to finalize the proposal?
- What does it mean to prepare the proposal now as the basis for documenting your completed project?

Use the Practice Scholarship Applications (at the end of this chapter) to help document your learning from concept to competency, including relevant American Association of Colleges of Nursing (AACN) *Essentials* (2021).

As you finalize your proposal, you are striving to become precise in your language to make sure your readers understand clearly what you mean. As clinicians advance their education and their standing in the healthcare arena, professionally written communication becomes an even more important tool. Project proposals have applications in many arenas and underscore the value of this professional document. The previous chapters have focused on the content that should be included in a proposal. This chapter finalizes planning for the professional proposal document. It involves tailoring the writing to the professional audience. It also includes strategies for continuing the ideas and plans into the next phase of project implementation and thinking ahead about how the project results and discussion will be conveyed after the project is completed.

## QUALITY IMPROVEMENT ALERT

The main goal of clinical projects is quality improvement (QI). Use the content in this chapter to complete your QI clinical project proposal.

## REVISING THE FIRST DRAFT

Clear communication is central to scholarly work. Often, people write things they think are perfectly clear, but then realize the information is clear only to them—clarifying the wording so others understand is key. Although the initial drafts are a matter of "getting it down in writing" and making it clear to yourself, the final draft is about making written communication clear to others. This means reflecting on the current draft (what has been produced or written) and what still needs to be done to finalize the proposal. It includes the use of precise language and maintaining consistency with terms to make sure your reader can understand and easily follow your meaning. Communication models support sending clear messages that others can interpret and respond to via feedback.

## COMPLETING THE FINAL PROPOSAL: QUESTIONS TO GUIDE YOUR WRITING

The hallmark of completing the proposal is paying attention to all of the details, including the proposal substance, structure, appendices, and writing and editing. Your table of contents can serve you well in organizing your narrative and provides good direction for you and your readers. Suggested questions to guide proposal completion are included in the following sections.

### Proposal Substance

Conveying important content that helps enhance your project proposal is key. Make sure you have addressed the following:

- Is the project purpose important in helping care for or benefit your population of interest?
- Is the proposal purpose statement clearly written and consistently restated throughout the proposal?
- Are the three triangle anchors—purpose, methods, and outcomes—consistent throughout the proposal?
- Have summaries been used to repeat key section ideas for reader clarity?

### Proposal Structure

Writing a proposal that meets scholarly criteria for communicating with other professionals is key. Are the following proposal sections clearly identified and written in scholarly format?

- introductory section, which clarifies the project problem and purpose
- review of the literature
- method section

### Proposal Appendices

The appendices must be complete and referred to in the narrative. Be sure to include

- the data-collection tools and any needed permission forms, if using developed copyrighted tools;
- agency agreements to complete the project;
- any needed institutional review board (IRB) and human subjects' approvals; and
- any consent forms (approved format).

### Writing and Editing

Self-editing is an early step in finalizing your proposal. The following basic guides can provide a useful starting point:

- Has the approved writing style (such as that of the American Psychological Association [APA, 2020]) been used correctly and consistently?
- Has clear wording been used?
- Has a consistent tense been used throughout?
- Have terms and abbreviations been appropriately introduced and referred to consistently throughout?
- Have headings been used to their best advantage to help outline the content and facilitate smooth flow of content? These headings link the proposal parts together, provide cues for the reader, and keep the reader moving forward.
- Has all cited work been referenced appropriately?

## ADDITIONAL WRITING TIPS

Clear expression of your message is key. Further tips for clarifying your written proposal include the following:

- *Avoid excessive use of acronyms and avoid confusing abbreviations*: For example, if you are referring to mental illness as "MI," medical-surgical nurses will immediately think about myocardial infarction. Again, be sure all abbreviations are properly introduced per your respective writing-style guidelines.
- *Use appropriate terms appropriately (do not mix concepts)*: Define the terms you will be using in the initial sections of the proposal. For example, "simulation" is sometimes used to indicate use of standardized patients and other times to describe high-fidelity technology-supported simulation. Be clear about what you mean.
- *Stay consistent with key terms*: Do a final "search" on the main terms (and any that you have described as interchangeable) and make sure they are consistent in all sections of the proposal. Go back and see what terms you used early on and confirm consistent use throughout the proposal.

- *Use summary statements*: Summary statements can be powerful in tying parts of a proposal together.
- *Use scholarly language and be precise in methods language*: Be careful to use the right term; for example, do not mix up the terms *content validity* and *content analysis*.
- *Seek consistency in lists*: Items should include consistent phrasing. For example, if the first item in a list uses an "ing" phrase, then all successive items in the list should be written in the same way (e.g., *caring, coupling,* and *changing*).
- *Punctuate*: Make sure that sentences are not too long and hard to follow. Can you read each sentence aloud and still breathe at the end?
- *Keep paragraph lengths appropriate*: Paragraphs that are too short lead to abrupt, choppy reading. On the other hand, paragraphs that are too long or that create a "wall of words" are hard to follow and lose the reader's attention. So, it is best in general to keep paragraphs to a minimum of three sentences and be sure to end paragraphs and start a new one as new topics or ideas are discussed. If you note a page-long paragraph, look for a place to break the paragraph into shorter paragraphs.
- *Write using the recommended style*: Although there are a variety of writing styles and you should use whatever you have been directed to follow, APA is the style often used in nursing. The style guidelines will direct all aspects of your final written proposal. For example, the use of third-person format is the typical scholarly format. If the first person is preferred, check first with your reviewing source/agency for appropriateness and then follow the APA guidelines in doing so.
- *Read the full project draft*: This helps you gain the big picture; you can then focus on needed details (Galvan & Galvan, 2017). Take this a step further and read the full proposal aloud, as this helps find sentences that don't flow well or phrases that don't make sense.

## FINALIZING THE TIMELINE AND PROJECT BUDGET

If not previously addressed in the proposal, now is the time to consider the project timeline and budget. These are two valuable components that keep a project moving forward.

### What Is the Project Timeline?

Although you have been thinking tentatively about a timeline for your project, this is the time to finalize it. As you return to your project map, consider what needs to happen when. List out each component of the proposal requiring an action and generate the best estimate of a time frame for each. One of the benefits of using Word tables or Excel spreadsheets is that they help you stay on track and communicate your plan clearly to others. You might add a little cushion to the timeline, as the time required for some activities (such as the institutional review board process) is often out of your control.

### What Is the Project Budget?

Although you have been thinking tentatively about a budget for your project proposal, now is the time to finalize this essential element. Some clinical projects will have minimal budgets that are subsumed as part of the work contribution to a setting. Sometimes there will be costs for things such as preparing surveys and/or providing snacks for participants. Consider and note these items.

If the proposal is being submitted for some type of grant funding, the project budget will be large enough to require a specific budget and budget justification. Excel spreadsheets can assist in clearly documenting and justifying the budget.

## TOOLS THAT FACILITATE PROPOSAL COMPLETION

### The Project Team and Committee

Recall that you have developed a team or committee to support you through the clinical project process. Just as the patient is part of their own clinical team, you are an important part of your project team. Once you have thoroughly reviewed and edited the proposal, seek your team or committee's review and use their time wisely. Similarly, if you took earlier advice and found a mentor, seek that person's review and feedback as well.

### Peer Review

Peer or colleague review of your proposal can complement team and mentor reviews. Seeking input and feedback from others who work with similar situations or topics can be invaluable, as it offers another objective review. The review provides an opportunity for further dialogue and more questions. If you serve as a peer reviewer, remember your role includes providing feedback that gives direction as well as offering encouragement and support to your colleague. Benefits of providing peer review include gaining critical-appraisal skills, participating in an interactive process, and practice at providing constructive feedback (Boehm & Bonnel, 2010).

With the opportunity of gaining peer or mentor feedback also comes the responsibility of receiving constructive feedback, reflecting on it, and responding to that feedback (Leedy & Ormrod, 2019). For example, working with mentors in finishing the proposal involves clear communication and responding to feedback on schedule. It also includes being mindful and respectful of others' time.

## Self-Review and Your Decision Trail

Reflection can provide both a proposal review and a debriefing of the proposal experiences. As a proposal review, reflective self-assessment against a standard, such as a proposal rubric, can be a helpful tool for self-accountability. Proposal rubrics, such as those provided in courses or from clinical agencies, serve as a type of guide. This reflective self-assessment can help examine your progress prior to submitting it to a mentor for feedback.

Reflection can also serve as a type of debriefing, allowing you to name what you are doing and learning. As you continue your reflective writing and decision trail, remember to write about not only what you are doing, but what barriers you have, how you deal with these, and general thoughts and impressions about how first the proposal, then the project, are progressing. Make an effort to extend this experience to include a weekly reflection on your work. The ongoing reflective decision trail serves as a written reflection to help document the project process and analysis. This can be useful as you later write up the final project, serving as a record of thoughts on the implementation process as well as emerging data. Opportunities are gained to focus on and facilitate project learning and to promote QI for future projects.

## REFLECTING AND SELF-EDITING

Complete a final self-edit as you read your final proposal draft out loud. That's right, read the draft proposal out loud, as you will be surprised at what errors—like those that get past the spell-check feature—slipped by when you were merely reading the words in your head. Are the following concepts evident?

- Does the challenge or problem grab and convince you within the first page?
- Are precise, consistent words used to describe key concepts?
- Are unnecessary adjectives deleted, such as *extra-special*?
- Is the third-person voice maintained throughout (or first person if acceptable via guidelines)?
- Are perfected grammar and spelling in place?
- Are abbreviations or acronyms used only minimally, if at all?

As you move forward with your clinical project, you will continue to exercise and strengthen skills that have helped you get to this point. Assets, such as accountability and goal setting, will serve you well in finalizing your proposal and moving to the implementation phase of your clinical project. Here are some points to follow to help in being accountable and to further goal setting:

- Ask relevant questions of your committee or team and use the feedback.
- Avoid the blame game when there are challenges to overcome.
- Work at problem-solving.
- Recognize strengths and limitations of a project.
- Continue your decision trail.

## PRESENTING YOUR PROPOSAL FROM THE PODIUM

In some cases, an oral presentation of the project proposal is required, either to a committee or a broader audience. As with the written proposal, you will want to communicate to others that your project proposal is based on a good idea, uses good evidence, and demonstrates sound approaches that others might replicate.

You will want to get the attendees' attention, helping them see the importance of the problem and that it needs to be addressed. You will share your proposal, then at a later date, you will share your finished project. This will include thoughts on why you pursued this project, what you did, what happened, what the outcomes were, and the "now what" components.

Your verbal proposal, often guided by a PowerPoint presentation, will address the who, what, where, and when of your proposal plans. Even if individuals have read a printed version of the proposal, the verbal presentation provides an opportunity to remind and focus participants on the key components. A sample format for proposal slides for a PowerPoint presentation is provided in Exhibit 15.1. This sample presentation contains content to be included in the presentation, a logical order for that content, details needed on each slide, and a sample narrative to accompany your slides. Follow this template (or others provided by your program) and you will have a thorough and well-organized proposal presentation.

## NEXT STEPS: USING THE PROPOSAL FOR PROJECT IMPLEMENTATION AND FINAL REPORT WRITE-UP

Although this book is about proposal writing, providing a hint regarding what is to come in the next project phases is appropriate. Once the hard work of pulling together multiple pieces of your proposal is accomplished and approved, the next steps involve project implementation and evaluation, writing the final report, and continuing scholarly plans for project dissemination. Project implementation is discussed in Chapter 16, which provides guidance on how to navigate the actual completion of your proposed project. During this time, you can also prepare to use your proposal to document your final written report, which is discussed in Chapter 17.

An important long-term goal for the proposal is that it be used as the basis for documenting the completed project. In

> **EXHIBIT 15.1 SAMPLE FORMAT FOR A POWERPOINT PRESENTATION OF THE PROPOSAL**
>
> The following sample slides for a "created" clinical project proposal follow a basic abstract format and might serve as a template or at least help generate ideas for a PowerPoint presentation of your proposal. Remember to use short, bulleted content on your slides, and then fill in the details with your narrative.
>
> **Slide 1:** *Title:* New Graduate Perceptions of Readiness to Use Electronic Health Records
>
> *Author:* W. Brown
>
> **Slide 2:** Thanks to committee members...
>
> **Slide 3:** *My background:* As a DNP student on a clinical leadership track, I really enjoy working with new graduates in my clinical specialty area and hope to guide them in projects such as use of electronic health records (EHRs).
>
> **Slide 4:** *What brought me to this project:* I was concerned by the number of challenges I was seeing when new graduates reached the clinical setting related to EHRs. EHRs are relatively new, but they are key to patient safety and interdisciplinary communication.
>
> **Slide 5:** *What was the purpose:* The purpose of this project was to survey graduating students on their perceptions and perceived readiness to use EHRs.
>
> **Slide 6:** *Brief literature review:* I found some medical literature about beginning graduate student use of EHRs but very limited studies were available in nursing or other disciplines. The most valuable studies were...
>
> **Slide 7:** Methods
> - This will be a descriptive survey administered at one setting.
> - Graduating seniors will be surveyed at a final class session.
> - Consent for the study will be attained by the school's human subjects committee.
>
> **Slide 8:** The survey
> - The surveys to be used are adapted from the EHR Survey and Brief Demographic Data Tool (Bonnel, 2011).
> - The Bonnel (2011) EHR Survey was adapted from two descriptive surveys in the literature.
> - The EHR Survey has two open-ended questions and 12 closed-ended items for participant rating, using a 1 (*low*) to 4 (*high*) scale.
> - A sample item is "I am adequately proficient in EHR skills."
> - The survey will be pilot tested with three junior nursing students to support clarity.
>
> **Slide 9:** Methods
> - A letter of invitation to the graduates along with the surveys will be provided to all graduating seniors at the close of one class.
> - All surveys will be collected in a large box by a second faculty member.
>
> **Slide 10:** Analysis
> - Descriptive statistics for *demographic* data will be completed and a table of descriptive sample characteristics created.
> - Descriptive statistics for *closed-ended survey items* will be completed and a summary table created.
> - Common themes from the content analysis will be identified from *open-ended responses* and exemplars provided.
>
> **Slide 11:** Project strengths/limitations
> - Strengths include the benefits of gaining graduates' perceptions via survey data.
> - Limitations include the fact there is just one sample and one setting and they may not represent the full graduate population.
>
> **Slide 12:** Potential project implications
> - *For practice:* Gaining new graduates' perceptions of EHR knowledge may lead to ideas for orienting new graduates in EHR use.
> - *For education:* Further education may be recommended in the student setting.
> - *For further research:* Further study of the best ways to learn and use EHRs may be indicated.
>
> **Slide 13:** Thanks to the committee, and thanks to audience members for their interest.
>
> **Slide 14:** Questions?

most cases, using the proposal as a component of the final project involves changing the verbiage from the future tense (used in the proposal) to the past tense (after the project has been completed). Clarifying details of the actual project implementation are added. Remember the review of literature is ongoing throughout the entire project, and you need to be sure it is updated to reflect the most current literature on your topic. The results, discussion, and implications sections are then added to these initial proposal sections to complete the final report. Consider laying out sample blank tables now while awaiting your data and analyses. Similar changes are also made to the project abstract, where the tense of proposal content is changed from future to past tense, and results and discussion content are added. It is not too soon to give thought to your project implementation and final analysis and write-up by thinking about this content now.

Also, learn from the experience of DNP students who have completed proposals. Their advice is presented in the Advice From DNP Students box.

### ADVICE FROM DNP STUDENTS

**Finalizing Project Writing**

Create your proposal in parts and seek feedback on each part.

- Receiving feedback on the parts (or sections) prior to completing the full task is very helpful.

Be prepared for multiple revisions.

- Numerous revisions are normal, even for people who have been doing this for a while.

Allow time for edits and rewriting.

- The proposal process contains many revision stages.
- The rewriting is very time-consuming; I kept thinking, "Gosh, I hope I am getting closer to a proposal."
- I learned why it was necessary to reevaluate and rewrite, and rewrite and rewrite.

Keep referring back to the project triangle.

- The most important thing that I learned while completing my proposal was always to refer back to my project triangle to stay focused.

There is no such thing as a perfect paper.

- Put ideas on paper as best you can; then consult your mentor.

### PRACTICE SCHOLARSHIP APPLICATIONS

Consider your competency documentation plans. How will your project address select *Essentials*? Consider additions to your project notebook as you complete the following.

- *Concepts to competence*: Think about your knowledge of writing professional documents. What questions do you have? How will you prepare your document as a cohesive whole, rather than separate pieces stuck together? How will you use your proposal to facilitate completion of your final clinical project report?
- *Essentials*: Review all of the advanced level competencies and subcompetencies (4.1, 4.2, and 4.3) in the Scholarship for Nursing Practice *Essential* domain. Reflect on how your project work addresses each.
- *Project notebook*: Self-assess your progress with the work outlined in this chapter, including identification of your strengths and areas for improvement.

## SUMMARY AND KEY POINTS

The proposal serves as a valuable communication tool, necessitating clearly written communication that is central to scholarly work. Completing the proposal involves gaining better writing skills, the goal being not only planning project methods, but also clearly conveying them. The value of gaining new tools for writing and completing the clinical project proposal, as well as reflecting on what has been accomplished, is a part of this. Considering next steps in implementing the proposal helps move toward project completion and contributes to quality patient care outcomes. Start preparing for documentation of your final project now by thinking about the results and discussion sections of your final paper, as well as the final abstract. Points to recall from this chapter include:

- In your review of the final proposal document, include attention to the proposal substance, structure, and appendices, as well as editing.
- Avoid common editorial mistakes, such as confusing abbreviations, using incorrect or inconsistent key words, lack of summary statements, lack of scholarly language, using lists with inconsistent initial phrasing, and using APA format incorrectly.
- If not yet done, finalize the project timeline and budget.
- Be accountable for your own reflection and self-review.
- Along with your own work, draw on support and feedback from your project team or committee, mentor, and peer reviewers.
- Consider that any proposal presentation must be complete and organized, with professional slides to accompany your narrative.

## NEXT CHAPTER UP

How do you move forward now that your project proposal is done and your proposal has been approved? How do you move forward to implement the plans presented in the proposal? What next steps exist for using your proposal to facilitate project implementation? The next chapter helps you address these questions.

### ONLINE/CLASSROOM DISCUSSION

In discussions with your colleagues, share responses to the following:

- You have now completed your clinical project proposal. Discuss what it means to have a professional and scholarly document. What questions do you still have about writing a professional and scholarly document? What have you learned in the process of writing your clinical project proposal?

## LEARNING ACTIVITIES

### Peer Feedback

When reviewing colleagues' proposals as part of peer review discussions (online or face to face) consider the following questions:

- As a reviewer, what do you think works well with this project?
- What concerns or further thoughts do you have about how this project is set up?
- What additional ideas do you have to help support the project success?

### To-Do List

A final proposal check:

1. Is the full proposal document packaged professionally as a scholarly document? Does it follow a systematic approach? Appropriate metrics? Reasonable analysis plans? Do you have plans for tables and graphs to clearly convey future findings?
2. Has your proposal undergone peer review (by colleagues, your mentor, and the project team)?
3. Have you written summaries of each proposal section for clarity? Is the finished proposal written in scholarly format?

## REFERENCES

American Psychological Association. (2020). *Publication manual of the American Psychological Association* (7th ed.).

Boehm, H., & Bonnel, W. (2010). The use of peer review in nursing education and clinical practice. *Journal of Nursing Staff Development*, *26*(3), 108–115. https://doi.org/10.1097/NND.0b013e3181993aa4

Bonnel, D. (2011). *Physical therapist assistant students' attitudes towards electronic health records* [Unpublished senior project]. Washburn University.

Galvan, J. L., & Galvan, M. C. (2017). *Writing literature reviews: A guide for students of the social and behavioural sciences* (7th ed.). Routledge.

Leedy, P., & Ormrod, J. (2019). *Practical research: Planning and design* (12th ed.). Pearson.

# SECTION IV

## Finalizing Your Proposal and Project: Next Steps

# 16. Moving the Proposal to Completed Project

## INITIAL THOUGHT

"Nursing is all about patient care, so a good project that helps improve the quality of care makes sense."

## CHAPTER CONTENT

- Reflective Questions
- Quality Improvement Alert
- Using Strategies From Quality Improvement to Implement Your Project
    - Common Assumptions in Implementing a Quality Improvement Project
    - Revisiting Your Proposal Protocol
    - Adhering to Project Procedures as You Implement Your Proposal
    - Potential Implementation Issues: The Setting/Context
- Implementation and Project Management
    - Engaging the Team
    - Scheduling Specific Project Components
    - Pilot Testing the Implementation and Data-Collection Procedures
    - Revisiting Project Evaluation Data
    - Continuing Professional Communication With Team Members
- Evaluating Your Final Protocol Implementation
    - Staying Within Your Budget
- Practice Scholarship Applications
- Summary and Key Points
- Websites for Further Review
- Next Chapter Up
- Online/Classroom Discussion
- Learning Activities
    - Elevator Speech
    - Organizational Support Network

## REFLECTIVE QUESTIONS

In Chapter 15, you completed your written proposal, not only planning project methods and outcomes, but also gaining better writing skills to clearly convey them. In this chapter, you have the opportunity to further review your skill set to be able to implement your project. With which of the following reflective questions are you the most confident?

- Adhering to your project protocol (your proposal) to carry out what you have said you will do?
- Working professionally with team members in leading projects?
- Using change-management principles to promote project implementation, evaluation, and enduring project results?

Use the Practice Scholarship Applications (at the end of this chapter) to help document your learning from concept to competency, including the relevant American Association of Colleges of Nursing (AACN) *Essentials* (2021).

## QUALITY IMPROVEMENT ALERT

Moving a quality improvement (QI) project to implementation can have similarities to other types of projects. The focus of a QI project includes a systems-based approach and increased emphasis on change models as ways to partner with the clinical agency.

A successful proposal gets you to the exciting part of your project: the actual implementation and evaluation. Your proposal has been approved by all required committees and ethics review boards. You have your purpose, you have your methods, and you have named the outcomes you will evaluate. Now what?

You now have a commitment to follow your project protocol. Your proposal is a type of ethical agreement that states you will do what you have said. It also allows opportunity for others to know what you have done and to critique and learn from this. If, for example, you have an evidence-generating project, such as a large needs assessment to learn of and document a chosen population's challenges, others will want to know your process for reaching the conclusions you did. As you move forward to this implementation phase of your project, major components include adhering to project protocols, continuing professional team communications, and following general project management processes.

## USING STRATEGIES FROM QUALITY IMPROVEMENT TO IMPLEMENT YOUR PROJECT

Although there are diverse approaches to implementing projects, QI is very common and has been chosen as a sample approach for this chapter (Table 16.1). Common assumptions and the importance of the project protocol follow.

## Common Assumptions in Implementing a Quality Improvement Project

- An evidence-based QI project involves implementing the best evidence as a protocol in one specific setting. Its particular value is in the application of evidence to improve a specific setting and/or population problem.
- Application of an evidence-based protocol to a specific setting is done to achieve select improved outcomes. Models that guide this type of project are typically QI models that incorporate systems theory and change theory.
- The particular value of QI is the outcomes achieved by the application of an evidence-based protocol to a specific setting. Although QI projects are not intended to be generalized beyond the context of the setting and

**TABLE 16.1 SAMPLE PROTOCOL CONSIDERATIONS TO GUIDE PROCEDURE SETUP USING A SYSTEMS APPROACH OF STRUCTURE, PROCESS, AND OUTCOMES**

| | Example: Implementing a Basic Fall-Prevention Plan | |
|---|---|---|
| **QI Component** | **Points to Consider** | **Time Frame** |
| **Structure/Process**<br>Education procedure for fall-prevention protocol | Include the who, where, what, and when:<br>• Who will deliver? How to deliver?<br>• For what audience? Where?<br>• When will staff receive the protocol?<br>Format: Builds on adult education theory<br>Sample strategies include: Face-to-face staff development session; building on staff knowledge using pretest about factors important in fall prevention; making the project relevant to the unit by including documented needs, concerns, and case examples | Create a timeline for education procedure. |
| **Structure/Process**<br>Resource development for fall-prevention protocol, including:<br>• Patient fall-risk assessment form<br>• Room safety scan tool<br>• Prevent-falls form for staff | Implementation resource development:<br>• Resource tools developed, reviewed, and organized<br>• Handouts of tools readily available for staff review (including electronic versions available)<br>• Ongoing visual cues as unit project reminders<br>• Project discussion opportunities at scheduled staff meetings<br>Create positive environment for the change and opportunities to promote success. Prepare needed resources and technology as directed on the timeline. | Create a timeline for resource development and electronic accessibility. Include sequencing of specific tasks |
| **Outcomes**<br>Evaluation of fall-prevention plan | Implement the evaluation plan and gain outcome data, including:<br>• Staff intent to use plan resources<br>• Staff knowledge gain and satisfaction with the educational presentation<br>• Patient unit fall numbers (during designated periods)<br>• Benefits to the organization (e.g., quality care and cost savings with improved care processes) | Create a timeline for data collection with each of the noted outcomes |

population, they should be clearly described so others can replicate and test them within their own settings and populations.

- Clearly naming and describing your implementation plans (the recipe or protocol you will follow) provide potential for others to replicate the project in a different setting.

- Further learning opportunities about QI approaches are available such as those provided by the Institute for Healthcare Improvement (IHI): www.ihi.org/resources/Pages/Tools/Quality-Improvement-Essentials-Toolkit.aspx.

## Revisiting Your Proposal Protocol

This chapter uses an evidence-based QI project on fall prevention as a protocol implementation example (Table 16.1). For those wanting to make a positive difference in healthcare, there is value in considering an evidence-based QI project (Melnyk & Morrison-Beedy, 2019).

Let us assume you have an approved QI proposal on fall prevention influenced by an evidence-based protocol (Agency for Health Care Research and Quality [AHRQ], 2013). You have completed your needs assessment as part of your preparation for project implementation. You have an engaged team that wants to work with you and you have worked with them to determine and develop the best evidence-based protocol. Now, for this unit QI intervention (your evidence-based fall prevention program), you will seek to implement your project successfully, evaluate outcomes, and share any lessons learned from your specific context or setting. You have laid out your proposal and have clear documentation of approved protocol procedures. Time to carry on.

## Adhering to Project Procedures as You Implement Your Proposal

It is important to clearly name and indicate how each project component is implemented (often there are multiple components or procedures that need to be specified within a project). Written project reports too often state that the project was implemented. Conn and Groves (2011) note that project directors decrease the impact of their interventions when they do not describe these fully. For example, let's say you named your project the Fall-Prevention Plan with your protocol procedure influenced by the AHRQ (2013) guides. Now you will be teaching staff about the project guides and have resources available to them. As you begin to implement these two project components, broad questions to address include asking yourself:

1. Have you made sure that staff support for the protocol has been gained?
2. Have you addressed how the protocol will be rolled out (including both structure and process components as well as a timeframe)?
3. Have you named who will deliver the educational sessions and who will have tool kit resources available?
4. Have you determined the education format for staff education about the protocol? Where/how will the educational sessions on the protocol be provided?
5. Have you addressed where and how staff will access the toolkit resources?

## Potential Implementation Issues: The Setting/Context

As you prepare for project implementation, it is essential that you clearly review your context, your team, and their readiness for the project. Review your proposal summary of relevant data and background information (the who, what, where, and when type issues) of your project context. As discussed in the earlier chapters, this includes people, resources, and processes. Confirm implementation readiness as described in the following:

- Have you addressed the context and setting of the organization (geographic location, rural/urban, clinical unit size, and structure); the people factors (patient population, staff/professional care team composition, staff numbers, relevant clinical specialties and educational preparation, and project relevant reporting structure of leaders and staff); and specific resource factors needed to support your project?

- Is site acceptance documented and readiness confirmed? Do you have a formal acceptance (such as an official letter) in your proposal? Have you completed the process of reminding both formal and informal agency members of acceptance of your project implementation (i.e., is there still support from senior leadership and any team members who will be involved with implementing the proposal)?

Why is description of the context so important at this point of implementation? One reason to clearly describe the context of the project is so others from diverse settings can perhaps benefit from the evidence-based plan you implemented. Since a QI project is typically not generalizable to other settings, others will have to consider their context and your project's relevance. In addition, you need to consider how your project context supports or detracts from your implementation.

## IMPLEMENTATION AND PROJECT MANAGEMENT

At this time, it is essential that you revisit your proposal preparation work and make sure your team is engaged in the implementation. Considerations for successfully implementing and maintaining change within broad change theory might include the concepts of engaging, scheduling, pilot testing, and revisiting.

## Engaging the Team

Your project team, those individuals who help implement the project or that the project impacts, can make or break the success of your QI project. The best team will ideally feel the project is important and want to know that their effort in implementing it is valued. For actual project implementation, ask yourself whether you have addressed team engagement in ways such as the following:

- Have you considered how an implementation committee might be formed with staff from your designated unit? Ideally, these individuals would be highly motivated toward the change implementation and could then be considered unit "change champions."
- Have you used an initial survey to gain the staff's current knowledge and attitudes toward the planned change?
- Have you considered a unit communication blitz with posters and e-mails helping all staff understand the when, where, and what of the change implementation?
- Have you presented the project and its progress as a standing agenda item at appropriate staff meetings, again with the intent of keeping people involved and informed?
- Have you included meetings with project stakeholders to gain support in implementing the change?

## Scheduling Specific Project Components

Detailed project scheduling is important to avoid potential implementation problems, so revisit and communicate your project timeline to appropriate individuals. Clearly communicating in early planning stages and sending reminders again before implementation can make a difference. You will want all team members to know what to expect. Does your timeline

- allow for needed project approvals;
- identify specific project tasks and sequence them as to when needed;
- make people aware of specific project dates and gain confirmation these will still work;
- minimize the risk of project problems, such as understaffing, at important points in the project; and
- identify clear project start-and-stop times relevant to team members (providing the team guidance as to when the implementation role is completed and the project moves toward ongoing stabilization)?

## Pilot Testing the Implementation and Data-Collection Procedures

Why do you want to pilot test your project procedures and data-collection tools? The main reason is that if there are going to be problems, it is better to fix them prior to the actual project implementation. Related to data collection, for example, in Chapter 10 a project protocol included an observational room-scan tool as a potential component of a fall-prevention project. As a new tool, the following testing and piloting were reported.

- *Content validity*: This was gained from the literature and expert reviews; from the literature, the items listed were common considerations in room safety and two nurses familiar with fall risk reviewed the tool for content validity.
- *Piloting the room-scan tool*: The room-scan tool was piloted on three rooms to help identify problems in wording of items. Minor edits were made based on this pilot test.
- *Equivalence*: This is a type of reliability in which two people gain the same results. For this tool, two nurses implemented the tool on three rooms and had strong consistency on room scores. This served as a pilot of the tool as well.

If unforeseen challenges should occur during project piloting, you need to communicate with your team about any needed protocol procedure changes and to confirm any alternate plans. Document these unexpected changes in the decision trail you are keeping. Consult with your committee chair to determine whether the changes are such that they need to be communicated to your institutional review board as well.

## Revisiting Project Evaluation Data

Various approaches, as previously noted, can be used to evaluate your project. QI models include evaluation concepts to remind us of this component. Referring again to the QI fall-prevention plan presented earlier in this chapter, how does your proposal direct you to evaluate the structure and process components of your protocol (including the face-to-face staff development session and the resources provided to staff)? In addition, as outlined in Table 16.1, consider how you will best document and organize designated outcomes such as staff intent to use project resources, staff knowledge gain and staff satisfaction with the educational presentation; patient unit fall numbers during designated periods; and benefits to the organization (such as better quality care and cost savings with improved care processes).

## Continuing Professional Communication With Team Members

Your proposal serves as a contract with your project committee and other team members. It provides the detail for keeping others on track (clarifying who will do what and when they will do it). Interprofessional team members should be included as there are benefits to incorporating the diverse perspectives multiple disciplines have to offer. Proposal implementation also involves meeting professional standards in working with the team, including clear communication and monitoring team function.

In making the most of your team, consider the following points for leading and engaging your project team members during the implementation phase:

- Confirm who is on the project team, including key team members and both formal and informal team members. Using a team network map to diagram central team members and other involved individuals can be useful.
- Be clear on naming and communicating the scope of the project to the team, including what it is and is not (via protocol).
- Help staff understand how the project fits the big-picture mission and goals of the organization.
- Be present at unit meetings and have an item on meeting agendas. Build on the current unit situation and show how the project can help improve or prevent problems.
- Conduct effective project team meetings that address good principles of leading meetings such as clear meeting agendas, responsibilities of team members assigned or volunteered, and clear follow-up minutes.
- Use good communication techniques, including active listening, questioning, and being present.
- If indicated, create team job descriptions for the project. Address how project duties fit with usual staff assignments.

## EVALUATING YOUR FINAL PROTOCOL IMPLEMENTATION

While you evaluate individual project components as they are carried out, and as you finish your implementation, it is important to take time to evaluate the full project implementation. Sample approaches include use of decision trails, reflective debriefing, and lessons-learned summaries.

*Decision trails with reflective logs*, as previously discussed, provide a summary of important activities (and their dates) that have been completed during project implementation This can serve as the basis of a report that allows others to see the structure and process you have used in implementing your project. Use of this method of documenting is one way to be sure that you are staying true to your protocol procedures. As you record factual dates and activities, include a reflective summary as a reminder not only of what is being done, but also why choices were made. This reflection also allows you to self-assess and address your satisfaction with the project accomplishments (i.e., highlighting the major accomplishments as well as noting what still needs to be accomplished). This can create a record for the final report as well as tips for future project work.

*Reflective debriefing* provides an additional approach to completing and learning from a project. Leading the team in reflection or debriefing about the completed project provides an opportunity to gain the team's perspectives. In a debriefing, the leader helps the staff address questions such as what happened, so what, and now what? Project debriefing can help address the actual facts of the situation, as well as emotional responses from the team. Sample questions you might ask as discussion leader include the following:

- What was the biggest challenge with the project?
- What worked well?
- What are opportunities for improvement?
- What surprises or barriers did the project team need to deal with?

As a component of the debriefing, you can summarize lessons learned in completing the project. A *lessons-learned summary* section documents your QI approach and promotes opportunity to improve approaches in future projects. It also promotes the quality of the project as a whole and can help document how organizational goals are being addressed and met through projects.

A final evaluative component is to review (check off) the points from your protocol. Sample points include asking yourself:

- Has your project stayed true to your protocol procedures as you completed interviews and surveys and guided discussion groups?
- Have you used guiding principles for ethical data collection?
- Have you addressed data security and analysis?
- Have you provided enough detail for the reader to replicate the project in a different setting?
- Have you stayed true to your full proposal as you summarized project analyses and results?

### Staying Within Your Budget

You want to determine the possible costs and benefits of your project. As you consider your project budget, a good budget plan addresses the required structure and process costs of your project. Creating or using an available budget template can serve you well. Keeping the project "in the black" and supporting positive outcomes is an obvious goal. As you review your budget, consider the following:

- Have you worked with your project team in clearly naming and sharing the outcomes target and budget that goes with it?
- Have you helped the team consider how the project fits the agency's mission and strategic plan?

- Have you included the budget as part of a larger benchmark-type document to check and make sure the project is staying on track? These documents work best if they include specific goals, dates, and people responsible. These score sheets or monitoring tools can be used to track costs in project goal attainment.
- Have you considered, appropriate in some projects, opportunities for reimbursement from outside sources to help offset project cost?

### PRACTICE SCHOLARSHIP APPLICATIONS

Consider your competency documentation plans. How will your project address select *Essentials*? Consider additions to your project notebook as you complete the following:

- *Concepts to competence*: What key tools have you gained for implementing your project? Review the questions from the beginning of this chapter and self-assess on your progress with this chapter as you begin your work.
- *Essentials*: Review advanced-level competencies and subcompetencies for the Knowledge for Nursing Practice, Scholarship for Nursing Practice, Quality and Safety, Systems-Based Practice, and Population Health *Essentials* domains and reflect on how they relate to your clinical project.
- *Project notebook*: Complete a one-page written reflection that considers your potential project implementation challenges and how you plan to address these.

## SUMMARY AND KEY POINTS

Your project implementation provides the opportunity to carry out what your proposal has promised. Key points include revisiting your proposal protocols and staying true to what you have said you will do. This chapter discussed a sample QI approach to implementation. Points to recall from this chapter include the following:

- Name and be consistent in project implementation procedures. For example, in a project with multiple components, such as evidence-based resource development and staff education, clearly describe and follow each.
- Review common assumptions for QI. Based on QI models, theses typically incorporate systems theory and change theory.
- Clearly address context issues, such as facilitators and barriers, that may impact your clinical project implementation.
- Carefully pilot test any project procedures and data-collection tools.
- Consider change-management principles that promote a project with enduring results.

- Address and follow your project budget.
- Review your approaches for professional communication and working professionally with team members.
- Evaluate your full project implementation with tools such as decision trails, reflective debriefing with staff, and lessons-learned summaries.

## WEBSITES FOR FURTHER REVIEW

- Health Resources and Services Administration (HRSA) programs and stakeholders:
  https://bhw.hrsa.gov/sites/default/files/bureau-health-workforce/funding/hrsa-pcte-toolkit-full.pdf
- Logic model based on systems components of structure, process, and outcomes (SPOs) and considers short, medium, and long term benefits:
  https://bhw.hrsa.gov/sites/default/files/bureau-health-workforce/funding/hrsa-pcte-toolkit-full.pdf
- Model AHRQ and Unit Safety Comprehensive Unit-Based Safety Program (CUSP) Program:
  www.ahrq.gov/hai/cusp/index.html
- AHRQ Team STEPPS:
  www.ahrq.gov/teamstepps/instructor/essentials/pocketguide.html
- Institute for Healthcare Improvement Quality Improvement *Essentials* Toolkit:
  www.ihi.org/sites/default/files/QIEssentialsToolkit.pdf

## NEXT CHAPTER UP

The next chapter describes writing up the final report of your project. The chapter includes opportunities for sharing or disseminating your project as part of an academic program.

### ONLINE/CLASSROOM DISCUSSION

You are planning to implement a patient education module on the *Speak Up* program. You have used a systems model to outline the structure and process resources available to you. Your outcomes of improved patient knowledge on this topic will be evaluated with a short true/false quiz. What is needed at this point to facilitate implementation on your clinical unit? What are you missing or still needing to know to ensure a successful roll-out of this project?

## LEARNING ACTIVITIES

### Elevator Speech

Elevator speeches provide a good start on naming what you do and sharing this with others. After filling out a big-picture project template or map, develop and share with course colleagues or unit staff an elevator pitch about your project topic/purpose and then the methods you will use to implement the project. Incorporate the three points of the project triangle (purpose, methods, and outcomes). Self-check your elevator speech for clarity and brevity. Are you clearly naming the problem that your project helps to solve? Can others follow the methods you will use?

## Organizational Support Network

Prior to implementing a QI project, you will want to consider available organizational support systems and resources. What does your organization have in place for ongoing QI and clinical scholarship? Review and describe resource networks (include graduate-prepared nurses and/or interprofessional leaders) that could be available to you and your colleagues for project work and advising. If networks are not available to you in the agency, identify those in the broader community or appropriate national resources who might fill this need. How might you approach or engage with this group?

## REFERENCES

Agency for Health Care Research and Quality. (2013). *Preventing falls in hospitals: A toolkit for improving quality of care.* https://www.ahrq.gov/patient-safety/settings/hospital/fall-prevention/toolkit/index.html

Conn, V., & Groves, P. (2011). Protecting the power of interventions through proper reporting. *Nursing Outlook, 59*(6), 318–325. https://doi.org/10.1016/j.outlook.2011.06.003

Melnyk, B. M., & Morrison-Beedy, D. (2019). *Intervention research and evidence-based quality improvement: Designing, conducting, analyzing, and funding* (2nd ed.). Springer Publishing Company.

# 17. Moving the Proposal to Written Final Report

## INITIAL THOUGHT

"Completing the final written report is easier if you start with a strong proposal."

## CHAPTER CONTENT

- Reflective Questions
- Quality Improvement Alert
- From Idea to Completed Project
- Converting the Project Proposal to a Final Written Report
- New Sections in the Final Report
  - The Results Section
  - The Discussion Section
    - Relating Your Findings to the Project Purpose
    - Tying Results to the Initial Literature Review
    - Identifying Implications of Your Findings
    - Addressing Project Strengths and Limits
- Using the Project Abstract as a Tool to Finalize Your Work
- The Edit-and-Revise Process, Again
- Planning to Present Your Final Report
- The Project Notebook in Furthering the Final Project Write-Up
- Practice Scholarship Applications
- Summary and Key Points
- Websites for Further Review
- Next Chapter Up
- Online/Classroom Discussion
- Learning Activities
  - To-Do List

## REFLECTIVE QUESTIONS

Once you have implemented your clinical project, you turn to documenting what you have done. As you write the final report, you will pull the project proposal together with the results of your completed project. Again, there is a benefit in reflecting on your goals. Have you proposed and implemented a tight, strong project? Have you stayed true to your proposal? The following reflective questions will help you consider your plan to move forward. Which of the following do you have the most confidence responding to?

- Are you comfortable reflecting on what has been accomplished to date, including project implementation?
- Are you able to consider next steps in documenting the completed clinical project?
- Have you considered next steps in writing the final report?

Use the Practice Scholarship Applications (at the end of this chapter) to help document your learning from concept to competency, including the relevant American Association of Colleges of Nursing (AACN) *Essentials* (2021).

## FROM IDEA TO COMPLETED PROJECT

In the early chapters of this book, you considered what it means to write a scholarly project proposal. You started with a clinical problem and from that you developed a strong purpose statement. You searched the literature to help refine your purpose statement, place it into context, and establish the current state of the science regarding that problem. You used the literature to determine whether the appropriate approach to your project should be an evidence synthesis plus, evidence-based QI, or descriptive evidence-generating approach, and you identified a theory appropriate to guide that project. Additional time was spent addressing outcomes evaluation, the clinical project plan, the method section, credible clinical data, and the ethical aspects of your project.

When your project proposal was almost complete, feedback from multiple sources was sought and repeated revisions were made so that your proposed plans were communicated clearly to others in a professional and scholarly manner. You made sure the proposal plan addressed all three points of the project triangle such that you had a tight and consistent plan to serve as a road map as you implemented the proposed plan. With that implementation now completed, it is time to

## QUALITY IMPROVEMENT ALERT

The final write-up for a quality improvement (QI) project can have similarities to other types of projects. The focus for a QI report typically involves clarity of structure, process, and outcomes so that other agency staff can benefit.

document what you have done in the final project report so that it can be easily communicated to others.

## CONVERTING THE PROJECT PROPOSAL TO A FINAL WRITTEN REPORT

Scholarly proposals or papers share common features. (As noted, the term *project charter* is sometimes used to denote an abbreviated form of the proposal that focuses on the project action plan.) Common sections of your scholarly paper included the following:

- introduction with problem summary and purpose statement
- literature review
- project methods

With these sections already written in the proposal, the hard work on this content is already done and you can easily adapt them for the final report:

- *Introduction and method sections*: In your project proposal, these sections were written in future tense, because they described what you were going to do in the future. But now that you have completed these activities, go back to these sections and change the future tense initially used to past tense to show that you have now completed the work.
- *Literature review*: Keep in mind that the literature review is an ongoing process throughout the duration of the project. So, although you have the initial literature review that you wrote and synthesized, you should also have been continuing to search the literature and update your literature review section as you continued to work on your proposal and implemented the project. Go back and be sure that this section is up to date on the latest and most current literature.

## NEW SECTIONS IN THE FINAL REPORT

Using traditional scholarly paper sections, in addition to adapting and updating the original proposal sections (introduction, literature review, and method), your final report will include two new sections: results and discussion. Remember that the results section includes just the facts, presenting the data that were gained in an organized and meaningful way. The final section of a scholarly paper consists of the discussion and implications, where the findings are considered from the "so what" perspective. In both sections, as in the rest of the final report, be sure to use the table of contents to help organize the content. This helps keep you focused as you write about content with which you are very familiar and it helps readers follow and make sense of the content that is completely new to them. Be aware that while some graduate programs or agencies may request different formats or titling of sections, the same broad principles apply in naming results and implications.

### The Results Section

This section describes the results you gained from data collection. Build in the paragraphs that convey the results you obtained while implementing your project. No matter how you collected data—from interviews, surveys, observations, or document reviews—organize your information in a logical and accessible format for your readers.

If you have completed a qualitative, content analysis, for example, the results can be presented in paragraph form, with the different themes used as headings to guide both you and the reader in organizing and following the findings. Be sure to tie the identified themes to the actual data by giving specific examples (such as quotes from participants) that support each theme.

Quantitative data can often be presented primarily in table format to allow readers to review descriptive results and see the report's statistical analysis. Refer to each table in the narrative so that readers know where to find the data and analysis. The tables need to be clearly organized, so be sure to have rows and columns labeled well and in a manner that makes the analyses clear. Exhibits 13.1 and 13.2 provided sample table formats to get you started. Be sure the content in your tables is consistent with what you report in the narrative. Also, be sure to follow the guidelines of the *Publication Manual of the American Psychological Association,* Seventh Edition (American Psychological Association, 2020), which devotes an entire chapter to the use of tables and figures.

### The Discussion Section

The Discussion section serves as a type of commentary. It provides an opportunity to share your interpretation and opinions about your project findings as well as to discuss the implications of your findings. You will address these questions: What was accomplished by doing your project? What was gained from learning the specific results? The Discussion should also suggest to the reader what action should be taken and what should be done given these findings. Approaches include relating your findings to the project purpose and questions, tying results to the initial review of the literature, identifying implications or the "so what" of your findings, and describing strengths and limitations of the project.

#### *Relating Your Findings to the Project Purpose*

Relating your findings back to your purpose statement helps keep your findings focused. You also have the opportunity to relate project findings or outcomes to your initial theories and hypotheses.

## Tying Results to the Initial Literature Review

As noted, again plan to consider the literature and describe the similarities and differences found in your project results. This is the time to put your project findings into the context of the literature review.

## Identifying Implications of Your Findings

The "so what" approach to findings includes addressing current project implications for education and practice. The "what next" question can also be asked concerning future projects or research. This includes implications for your populations, patients, staff, and students.

## Addressing Project Strengths and Limits

Remind yourself to reconsider the strengths and limits of your completed project at this point and document these. A sample description of limits and strengths for a small QI project might include:

- *Limits*: Small descriptive sample results; tested in only one setting
- *Strengths*: Protocol developed from best-evidence literature; expert peer-review panel for protocol review

## USING THE PROJECT ABSTRACT AS A TOOL TO FINALIZE YOUR WORK

The project abstract will be the most read and beneficial document of your project, stating clearly and in limited space why the project was important, what was done in the study, and its outcomes and implications. Your abstract will include the key components of your proposal in abbreviated form. It can serve as a checklist that all important components of the project triangle (Appendix A) have been addressed. The abstract's abbreviated format also provides an easy communication tool for your team members. Note that the "proposal" abstract was a summary of the proposed project, whereas the "project" abstract is a summary of the completed project. A good abstract will demonstrate significance to practice, methodological soundness, and clear writing. Abstracts are generally limited in length—often to 100 to 150 words—so they need to be not only well organized, but also concise.

Just as your final report built on your proposal, the final project abstract builds on the proposal abstract. Revisit the proposal abstract and change the verbs to the past tense and fill in the project outcomes and implications. This revision of your initial proposal abstract addresses what work has been completed and highlights project results and their implications. Box 17.1 provides an example of a final project abstract. Your abstract should broadly answer the following questions:

---

**BOX 17.1 Final Project Abstract: Using Glucose Patterns to Improve Diabetes Management in Long-Term Care**

**Roberta Mansfield, DNP, APRN**

The LTC setting often provides systems-level challenges for both facility nurses and primary care providers who manage residents with diabetes. The purpose of this project was to outline the development of a diabetes management module that can be used as a facilitated training resource by staff nurses working in LTC, and to describe the impact of this intervention at the systems level. A 151-bed nursing care facility in the Midwestern region of the United States was the site for a QI project to educate 10 facility nurses on evidence-based practices for interpreting plasma glucose data, identifying trends and patterns, and communicating findings to providers. An instructional module was developed and piloted with nurse managers and staff nurses at the facility. A pre/posttest and module evaluation survey demonstrated positive acquisition of knowledge and skills related to the content at the time of implementation. A guided discussion session evaluated the sustainability of this intervention on individual clinical behaviors and their effect at the systems level. Through enhanced awareness and partnership with facility nurses, nurse practitioners will be better able to access and act on information essential to the improvement of glucose control for residents with diabetes.

LTC, long-term care; QI, quality improvement.

---

- Why did you begin the project?
- What specifically did you do?
- What did you learn?
- What are the implications?

To convert these questions into a scholarly communication format, the scholarly parts addressed in the abstract should include the following:

- *Context/background*: What was the setting and population? Why was this issue important? What was your purpose in doing this?
- *Brief literature*: What evidence did you find for the need/approach?
- *Method*: What did you do (systematic description)? How did you analyze/evaluate?
- *Results*: What did your data analysis find? What outcomes were produced?
- *Discussion and implications*: Why were the findings important to your populations? What are the implications for education, practice, and research?

## THE EDIT-AND-REVISE PROCESS, AGAIN

Recall the important lessons you learned along the way in completing your clinical project proposal. Of great importance right now is the content from Chapter 15 about reviewing, editing, and revising, which you now need to apply to your final report. Once again, you will want to check the paper for

- final report substance,
- final report structure,
- final report appendices, and
- writing and editing.

Again, this process requires your own accountability, as well as drawing on the feedback and support of your peers and project team. Be sure to seek and be open to constructive feedback—both positive and negative—from reviewers. The following tips are offered as you complete your final report electronically (Leedy & Ormrod, 2019):

- Save your document often.
- Use, but do not depend exclusively on, the spell-check and grammar features.
- Print out a hard copy for final proofreading.

Also, as suggested in Chapter 15, read that final hard copy aloud to help with final edits. Owens et al. (2020) provide helpful writing resources for students, including a general checklist for completing scholarly papers.

## PLANNING TO PRESENT YOUR FINAL REPORT

A scholarship of application suggests that a project is not complete until it is shared as a product. Prepare a clear and logically constructed PowerPoint presentation of your completed project, similar to your proposal presentation (discussed in Chapter 15). You will use some of the same slides as you did in your proposal presentation, including the project title, recognition of committee members, background, purpose, and literature review, although you will likely spend a little less time on each topic so that you have time to address the new content (results and discussion). Again, the tense used in your method section will be revised to past tense, and then you will add your results and discussion. Be sure the discussion places your results into the context of the most current literature, includes strengths and limitations of your project, and discusses implications for education, research, and practice. See Chapter 18 for guidance if your school requires a poster, rather than a podium, presentation of your final project.

## PROJECT NOTEBOOK IN FURTHERING THE FINAL PROJECT WRITE-UP

Your reflective project notebook documents your proposal journey and can be a major tool in furthering your project scholarship. Project notebooks provide an opportunity to package activities and name what you do in your clinical scholarship. It is a tool used to promote reflection and communication about accomplishments. A project notebook that documents each of the sections of your final report can showcase your ongoing clinical project progress and document one component of your clinical expertise. They also serve as a way to document clinical scholarship via naming and describing knowledge gained in your clinical project and supporting the generation of questions that require further study. The project notebook allows others to understand your work and provides potential that others could replicate it in their settings.

The reflective component of your project notebook, or a summary of your perspectives as to accomplishments and lessons learned, serves as a way to share your specific story about purposes and strategies for projects that advance safe, quality patient care. Your reflective project notebook helps you think about the big-picture process of your project as you complete the final project report and move on to considering dissemination of the findings within the broader profession (see Chapter 18). It also reminds you to address what surprised you, or what you would you do differently in a future project, essentially preparing you for the "what next?" The project notebook of your completed project helps support

- reflection on what you did,
- communication with others about what you did,
- ownership of the work and learning that has been accomplished,
- value in helping document this lengthy project, and
- organization for further project scholarship.

### PRACTICE SCHOLARSHIP APPLICATIONS

Consider your competency documentation plans. How will your project address select *Essentials*? Consider additions to your project notebook as you complete the following.

- *Concepts to competence*: What key tools have you gained for writing up your final project report? Review the reflective questions from the beginning of the chapter and self-assess on your progress with this chapter.
- *Essentials*: Review advanced level competencies and subcompetencies for the Systems-Based Practice, Knowledge for Nursing Practice, Quality and Safety, Systems-Based Practice, and Population Health *Essentials* domains and reflect on how they relate to your clinical project.
- *Project notebook*: Start with a one-page written reflection that addresses your project's final report. What do you anticipate as potential benefits and challenges to sharing your written implementation plan?

## SUMMARY AND KEY POINTS

Starting with a well-written proposal makes writing the final report easier. Minor edits to the background and method sections consist primarily of changing verbs from future to past tense. The original review-of-literature section must also be updated to include the most current literature on the project topic. Two new sections, results and discussion/implications, are then added to communicate the findings of your projects. The abstract is also updated with revised tense for appropriate sections and the addition of descriptions of your results and discussion. Points to recall from this chapter include the following:

- The initial sections of the final report come directly from the project proposal, with the tense changed from future to past.
- Two new sections are added in the final report: results and discussion/implications.
- The results section presents the data from your project in a meaningful way.
- The discussion section connects the findings to the project's purpose and places it in the context of current literature; identifies the project's strengths and limitations; and discusses the implications of the project for education, research, and practice.
- The traditional final report needs the same review and editing as was previously used to make the proposal a scholarly document.
- The project abstract is also updated with tense changes to early sections and the addition of results and discussion sections.
- The podium presentation of your final report will update your proposal presentation with new results and discussion sections emphasized.
- Project notebooks help document your application scholarship, clarifying your processes as well as the clinical products/outcomes.

## WEBSITE FOR FURTHER REVIEW

Some professional websites provide abstracts as well as completed DNP projects. An example includes the Doctors of Nursing Practice website with their Doctoral Project Repository: www.doctorsofnursingpractice.org/doctoral-project-repository/

## NEXT CHAPTER UP

Where do you go now that your final project report is completed and your podium presentation is done? How does your project move from a school's degree requirement to a project that truly impacts nursing practice? How do you disseminate your project findings so that they have a place in the scholarly body of literature that other professionals can access and use in their own practice? The next chapter helps you address these questions.

### ONLINE/CLASSROOM DISCUSSION

As you consider plans to share your clinical project, what are good publication venues to consider in your specialty? What ideas can you share with colleagues for publication venues for their project topics? Review a listing of nursing journals to gain additional ideas at the following website: https://airtable.com/app1QbygMN23wigqu/shrjqveaKHtS9xku8/tblNXTxmTr18CC1lf

## LEARNING ACTIVITIES

### To-Do List

A final report check:

1. Is the final report document packaged professionally as a scholarly document? Does it follow a systematic approach? Does the results section present the project data in a clear and meaningful manner? Does the discussion section connect the findings to the project purpose? Compare the findings to the most recent literature? Identify project strengths and limitations? Does it discuss the implications of the findings to quality care?
2. Have you written summaries of each final report section for clarity? Is the finished proposal written in scholarly format?
3. Has your final report been reviewed by peers (by colleagues, your mentor, and the project team)?

## REFERENCES

American Psychological Association. (2020). *Publication manual of the American Psychological Association* (7th ed.).

Leedy, P., & Ormrod, J. (2019). *Practical research: Planning and design* (12th ed.). Pearson.

Owens, J. K., Cowell, J. M., Kennedy, M. S., Newland, J. A., & Pierson, C. A. (2020). Mentoring the novice writer to publication: An update from the INANE student papers work group. *Nurse Author & Editor, 30*(3), 5. https://doi.org/10.1111/nae2.6

# 18. Moving Your Completed Project to Dissemination and Further Scholarship

## INITIAL THOUGHT

"If you are going to do a scholarly project, you really have a responsibility to share it."

## CHAPTER CONTENT

- Reflective Questions
- Quality Improvement Alert
- The Proposal and Project: Reflecting on What Has Been Gained
  - Clinical Scholarship Models
  - Clinical Scholarship and National Priorities
- Next Steps: Disseminating, Advancing, and Building on Your Project
  - Disseminating the Project via Varied Presentation Formats
  - Considerations for Abstract Preparations
  - Considerations for Verbal Presentations
  - Special Considerations for Poster Presentations
  - Planning for Publication
  - Proposals for Future Grant Writing
  - Proposals for Further Clinical Projects
  - Your Clinical Project Notebook and Your Career Portfolio
  - Wrapping Up Your Program
  - Career or Role Transitions
  - Further Mapping Out a Career Plan
- Additional Concepts of Value
  - Developing and Continuing the Mentor Partnership
  - Caring for Self and Having a Peer Group
- Practice Scholarship Applications
- Summary and Key Points
- Online/Classroom Discussion
- Learning Activities
  - Mentor Network Assessment
  - Continuing Project Self-Assessment and Reflection

## REFLECTIVE QUESTIONS

In Chapter 17, you focused on the writing skills necessary to complete your final written project, concentrating on how to clearly convey your project work. In this final chapter, you focus on the "what next" for your completed clinical project. The following reflective questions guide this chapter. With which of the following are you most confident?

- Are you ready to reflect on what has been gained in completing your proposal and project?
- Are you considering next steps in sharing and disseminating the completed project?
- Are you able to build on your DNP project as a contribution to future clinical scholarship?

Use the Practice Scholarship Applications (at the end of this chapter) to help document your learning from concept to competency, including the relevant American Association of Colleges of Nursing (AACN) *Essentials* (2021).

This chapter is about moving forward with sharing your project. It allows you the opportunity to stop and celebrate the accomplishment of creating a well-written project. It encourages you to reflect on the big picture of what has been learned in developing and completing this project and to reflect on what still needs to be done.

## QUALITY IMPROVEMENT ALERT

Dissemination for a quality improvement (QI) project can have similarities to other types of projects. The focus for QI dissemination is typically relevant to sharing project approaches with other relevant entities.

Your advanced clinical project has helped you name and focus an area of expertise. This chapter comes full circle in preparation for sharing this project and expertise. Using best practices for ongoing mentoring, peer review, and self-assessment will help to achieve your objectives. You will need to reflect on how to expand clinical scholarship and find opportunities for interprofessional team collaboration. Completing the project then leads to opportunities for disseminating your work and developing further projects.

## THE PROPOSAL AND PROJECT: REFLECTING ON WHAT HAS BEEN GAINED

### Clinical Scholarship Models

The AACN (2015) notes that all DNP students should implement a project that demonstrates clinical scholarship. The clinical project provides an opportunity to extend scholarship to the clinical setting. Clinical projects often relate to the scholarship of application. As noted earlier, Boyer (1990) described the importance of clinical or application scholarship in his classic scholarship framework.

The completed DNP project can demonstrate that you are accomplishing scholarly work and making a contribution to the profession as well as documenting competencies.

Through gaining proposal-writing and project skills, you have gained DNP graduate competencies, including methods to

- review and synthesize the best evidence for practice,
- develop projects to evaluate practice at varied levels from individual patient to populations and systems,
- use QI tools to enhance practice,
- use best evidence to guide protocol development to enhance patient care, and
- use technology to gain data to better understand the patient care process and outcomes and to generate further projects.

## Clinical Scholarship and National Priorities

Expanding clinical scholarship via the DNP project provides the opportunity to contribute to the profession. As previously noted, this clinical application scholarship has potential to help meet the changing needs of healthcare and help graduate students document clinical project competencies in the *Essentials* (AACN, 2021).

National initiatives, such as the Quality and Safety Education for Nurses (QSEN) program (Cronenwett et al., 2009) and the Institute of Medicine's (2003) Health Professions Education, provide broad direction as to important themes needed to achieve safe, quality care. Projects that address themes such as these contribute to clinical scholarship and the nursing profession's knowledge base. The following list summarizes themes within these resources:

- *Evidence-based practice*: The focus on evidence has been emphasized throughout this text. Reflect on how your project will help extend the use of evidence in practice. Consistent with guides for DNP scholarship, this is central to the work of all advanced practice nurses.
- *Technology*: Rapid advances in electronic health records and various clinical databases provide new opportunities for gaining data to better understand patient populations and their needs as well as to document clinical outcomes. Using technology to its fullest potential can include creative use of newer advances that facilitate both staff and patient interventions and data collection. Opportunities exist to gain data via provider, patient, and technology interfaces.
- *Collaborative work*: Optimizing the use of interprofessional teams is a central component of the agenda to improve healthcare. Teamwork included in team-supported clinical projects is an essential component of patient-centered care. Interprofessional competencies that include clear communication and scholarship have been developed to help move this effort forward (Interprofessional Education Collaborative, 2011).
- *Quality improvement*: The essence of advanced clinical projects is improving patient care quality. Clinical projects have the potential to lead to changes in systems that enhance quality and safety. In today's data-driven world, scholarly skills gained in proposal writing and project completion are key components for future lifelong learning and evidence-based practice.
- *Patient-centered care*: Opportunities exist to gain patients' perspectives of what quality care means to them. Focus on safety is a key component of relevant clinical projects as well.

## NEXT STEPS: DISSEMINATING, ADVANCING, AND BUILDING ON YOUR PROJECT

Your DNP project provides a good chance to learn dissemination skills and gain opportunities for continued clinical scholarship. It offers an opportunity to share the clinical value of the project specific to patient care, to the organization in which it was completed, and its value for further study.

When asking what counts as clinical scholarship, dissemination of scholarly work is a key component. According to Huber and Hutchings (2005), projects are considered scholarly when they are documented, peer reviewed, and passed on via public venues such as publications. Clinical projects can serve as a bridge to advanced clinical scholarship. Gaining the tools necessary to create scholarly presentations and publications provides the beginning of your further clinical scholarship journey. Completed projects can lead to

- presentations in varied formats (abstract, podium, webinar, and poster),
- future publications,
- proposals for future grant writing,
- opportunities for further clinical projects, and
- use of select components of the clinical project notebook as part of a career portfolio.

## Disseminating the Project via Varied Presentation Formats

Presentations provide opportunity for an audience to learn about your project accomplishments. Different DNP programs use different approaches to initial project dissemination. Some programs include both a proposal defense and a finished project presentation (both noted in Chapter 15). Once you have moved beyond your program presentations, common approaches for broad professional dissemination include abstract preparation, verbal presentations, posters, and publications. Although many of these formats have been done face to face in the past, many are now using virtual online formats for both verbal presentations and posters.

## Considerations for Abstract Preparations

Once you opt to share your project beyond your educational program, you will likely be submitting an abstract to be peer reviewed and, hopefully, accepted for presentation. Things to remember when submitting abstracts:

- Follow the abstract guidelines. Pay attention especially to any rubrics provided for reviewers. Before submitting, self-assess and determine how you would rate yourself and then fix any noted deficits.
- Follow the key sections of your project to organize your abstract. Note that usually there is a word-count limitation for abstracts.
- If submitting to a conference, try to relate your abstract to the conference theme or objectives, stating why this project is an important topic for this audience.
- Address the project implications and what the audience can gain (or how they might use this information in their own settings).
- Ask a peer colleague to review for clarity.

## Considerations for Verbal Presentations

Disseminating your project via presentation (whether via formal podium presentation or virtual webinar) provides opportunity to contribute your work to the profession. Tips for presenting your project via a verbal format include the following:

- Adhere to any presentation guidelines or templates provided by the specific program or organization.
- Know the basics: Who is your audience? When are you speaking? How long are you supposed to speak?
- As you develop a PowerPoint presentation or outline, begin by giving yourself credit. Include a slide with your credentials and experiences that guided you to the project.
- Thank your project mentors and acknowledge their work and guidance.
- Share your story; indicate why you chose to complete this project.
- To organize the presentation, follow the format of your project headings. Be concise, using bullets to convey the key facts and stay focused on your target information; limit extraneous information.
- Stay organized with PowerPoint slides that are easy to follow with needed visuals; use a reasonable number of slides.
- Use good public-speaking principles to introduce and finish the presentation (alert your audience via your introduction what you plan to tell them and end by summarizing what you told them).
- Engage listeners by building in appropriate questions or discussion points.
- Look professional and be professional in any communications relevant to these formal presentations.
- Have a back-up copy of your presentation available (i.e., e-mailed or thumb-drive copy).
- If you are presenting via real-time, online webinars, special considerations include checking connectivity issues and moving smoothly through the webinar system's mechanics. If you are new to this format, check if there is an opportunity for a practice session.

## Special Considerations for Poster Presentations

Why use a poster format to share your presentation? Posters offer the opportunity for people to quickly scan and learn about your project. Although historically posters have been shared in a face-to-face venue, now there are often opportunities for virtual or online poster presentations. Whether you are preparing a poster for a school dissemination day or professional meeting, tips for preparing posters include the following:

- Determine whether there are specific organization templates or guidelines to follow for the poster (some organizations have very specific guidelines).
- Make sure your project title conveys the "must-know focus" of the project for a specific audience (you may consider sharing different project components with different audiences).
- Start with an outline or PowerPoint format to guide your thinking (and logical ordering of content).
- Consider how best to achieve good organization and visibility. Focus on a clear presentation of important project components.
- Because not all project information will fit on a poster, sometimes an additional handout, for those seeking more detail, can be included that contains key points and references (you may want to share your e-mail for possible follow-up conversations).
- Whether in a face-to-face or virtual setting, try to engage participants with simple questions related to their interest or experience with the topic.

## Planning for Publication

Reasons to publish include sharing expertise, disseminating new evidence, gaining career advancement (in both education and clinical settings), developing your own knowledge and skills, and achieving your own satisfaction (Oermann & Hays, 2018). Those in diverse advanced clinician roles in particular have reason, even obligation, to disseminate the knowledge gained related to improving patient care. The next step for your project is writing your manuscript, changing it from academic format to publishing format. Format examples vary by the type of project selected and professional journal guides. Steps to help with the publication approach include the following:

- Create a timeline for publication (especially important as you finish your project).
- Determine the best journals for submission, considering the best audience for your project as you review the purposes of specific journals. Listings of journals and their areas of interest are available (at https://naepub.com.
- Revise your final paper to fit the journal's guidelines.
- Outline the manuscript, ideally immediately after a presentation, using your PowerPoint slides as your manuscript outline (changing from academic format to publishing format and following the journal's guidelines).
- For each diagram or table used, be sure to add a clear description, explaining it in the narrative; for example, sharing what different table rows and columns (relevant to your final project) mean.
- Just as you responded to faculty requests for revisions to your proposal and final project report, expect to receive reviewer requests for manuscript revisions. Try not to be discouraged. A request for revisions is a good sign there is interest in the manuscript.

## Proposals for Future Grant Writing

As advanced clinicians you will have future opportunities to write proposals and gain resources to document scholarship with populations of interest. In learning proposal-writing skills, you have also gained tools for critiquing and synthesizing the literature, creating worksheets for laying out the big-picture plans, and creating templates for mapping out future projects. Concepts used in proposal writing and in creating sections of proposals apply across most scholarly venues. You have gained a tool kit of resources to help document and make the case for future projects. The potential for grant funding exists with submission of well-written proposals.

## Proposals for Further Clinical Projects

Your initial project proposal often serves as a tool for learning and can serve as the basis for generating further projects. In considering future plans, recall that project proposals help communicate what you do as an advanced clinician and address further goal setting or "what's next?" with your specialty. As you move forward with doctoral scholarship, you may think about further projects to build your career and clinical specialty. Think about the following:

- Consider using your project proposal as a springboard for extending the topic.
- Consider using your completed project as a template for another project on a related topic.
- The project may lead to using similar project methods in further venues and to extending expertise with your specialty population.

Advanced clinicians have opportunities to practice with unique populations. These projects can help others better understand these populations and serve as tools for mentoring others.

## Your Clinical Project Notebook and Your Career Portfolio

A reflective *career portfolio* can make your projects and career activities easily visible and provide opportunity to document successes to share with others, as well as help learn from your challenges. Recall from earlier chapter discussions that the benefits of your *clinical project notebook* include helping document or track project components with other team members and sharing with others the scholarship that is developed in a clinical setting. The clinical project notebook also serve as a way to name and describe knowledge gained, as well as to support generating questions that require further study.

To begin or continue your career portfolio, create a three-ring binder or its electronic equivalent. Include new project summaries such as abstracts or brief project samples in addition to your DNP project activities. Career portfolios are most valuable when they also include your reflections as to why the projects and various components included are important. These reflections should include lessons learned and serve as a personal quality-improvement tool. Consider their benefit in situations such as wrapping up your program, transitions, and further career plans.

## Wrapping Up Your Program

As you come to the end of your DNP project and program, you are transitioning away from the support of your school and often creating a new role. The reflective career portfolio can help you acknowledge your program accomplishments. There is value in naming what you did and why, for both your own self-esteem and sharing with colleagues or faculty. Abstracts or brief samples from varied course assignments can help name what has been accomplished. As noted, your initial project notebook can also become an early chapter in your reflective career portfolio and a first step in sharing, presenting, and even publishing a successful project.

## Career or Role Transitions

Moving forward you will want to continue to maintain an ongoing career portfolio to serve as a collection of products with the potential to help name and clarify what you are doing as you move forward in your career. This can be beneficial, for example, if you are developing a new clinical specialty or career role and describing this to others. In some ways, the career portfolio becomes your personal book of accomplishments. This career portfolio, along with your curriculum vitae, can be used strategically to document career growth and stay on track with your career goals.

## Further Mapping Out a Career Plan

Often a career portfolio that has a reflective component can serve as a starting point for career mapping. As you review your portfolio, you can reflect on where you currently are in your clinical scholarship work and consider where you would like to be. For example, consider goals focusing on select components of common doctoral roles such as clinician, leader, and/or educator, maybe focusing on different roles during different career points and using the career portfolio to show the big picture of your career over time. Questions to guide you in mapping out your career portfolio choices (and ongoing work plans) include the following:

- Reflect on where you are today in your clinical scholarship. What are your strengths? Areas for continued improvement?
- Who are key people or mentors who have helped you develop clinical scholarship skills? Are there facilitators or barriers to reaching out to these people now?
- Reflect on your real-life clinical work situation with regard to scholarship. In your current work setting, what organizational factors support or detract from your ongoing clinical scholarship opportunities?
- What resources for mentoring or ongoing support does your clinical agency, community, or professional organizations (local, regional, or national) have in place that you can access to support ongoing scholarship?

## ADDITIONAL CONCEPTS OF VALUE

### Developing and Continuing the Mentor Partnership

Throughout the development of your project, you will be working with a mentor of some type.

In many cases, you will stay connected with faculty mentors after the project is completed. You may consider renegotiating future work with this person. Mentor and mentee roles may even coexist as you share your unique clinical expertise with your mentor in future projects. Additional possibilities include moving on to another mentor or considering whether you are ready to take on the mentoring role yourself. It is also likely you will gain informal mentoring from individuals related to your project, as well as from a more formal mentor. A mentor whose interests already match yours can provide a type of incentive to move forward. As described in Chapter 1, your mentoring relationship benefits from clear communication, both written and verbal. It should also involve fair, equitable use of the time of both mentor and mentee.

### Caring for Self and Having a Peer Group

Staying motivated to complete a big project involves caring for oneself. Remember to create time and space to care for yourself while focusing on your scholarship. This includes creating time and activities for physical and emotional health. Colleagues or peer groups can play a role in this process as well. Peers can help in debriefing project activities and help you stay motivated to complete your project. Peer groups can be formalized to include scheduled journal club–type activities or be maintained more informally.

> **PRACTICE SCHOLARSHIP APPLICATIONS**
>
> Consider your competency documentation plans. How will your project address select *Essentials*? Consider additions to your project notebook as you complete the following.
>
> - *Concepts to competence*: Appreciate your accomplishments in dissemination (as documented in your project notebook). Review the questions from the beginning of this chapter and self-assess on your progress.
> - *Essentials*: Review advanced level competencies and subcompetencies for the Knowledge for Nursing Practice, Schorlarship for Nursing Practice, and Quality and Safety *Essentials* domains and reflect on how they relate to your clinical project.
> - *Project notebook*: In a written reflection, complete a one-page dissemination plan. Once your project has been disseminated, add that summary/document as well.

## SUMMARY AND KEY POINTS

Being an expert clinician comes with the responsibility of clinical scholarship. You created a proposal for and then implemented a project of interest. Whatever your topic or approach, your work has been guided by the best evidence available as you considered the literature, theories, and models available. Your blend of knowledge, motivation, and the setting of your clinical project can lead to further scholarship as you finalize and then share your project with others. Once the proposal is implemented, and the final report written, the opportunity exists to further package and disseminate your learning to the broader professional community. Results of these important clinical projects then lead to developing practice improvements and help direct the future of patient care. Points to recall from this chapter include the following:

- Advancing your clinical scholarship is an important role for the DNP; your clinical project notebook can serve as a starting point for doing project dissemination.
- Clinical application scholarship via proposal competencies is a good fit with the DNP project and the AACN *Essentials*. National agendas, such as those developed by QSEN and the National Academy of Sciences, can help identify and support further needs for projects.
- Opportunities exist to disseminate your finished project professionally via varied formats, including abstracts, verbal presentations (face to face or webinar), and poster presentations as well as publishing opportunities in various journals.
- Your clinical project notebook, in concert with a reflective career portfolio can serve as the basis for ongoing scholarship as you build your clinical specialty.

### ONLINE/CLASSROOM DISCUSSION

Share and celebrate your completed project abstracts. Use this as a debriefing time to consider/share with your peer group: What has been accomplished? So what? And now what?

## LEARNING ACTIVITIES

### Mentor Network Assessment

Reflect on where you are in your career today. Consider your strengths as a clinical scholar. How would your colleagues describe you as a clinical scholar? Prompts to guide further reflection include the following:

- What type of mentoring do you need? Assess/identify the individuals you currently consider mentors and identify additional mentors you may need based on future professional leadership goals. Include mentors (or potential mentors) from your current work setting, broader community, and professional organizations (local, regional, and national).
- Based on your self-assessment, what goals will you set to enhance your clinical scholarship? What further mentorship will you seek?

### Continuing Project Self-Assessment and Reflection

Scholarship and mindful clinical practice go hand in hand. You have reflected on your work as you completed first the proposal and then the project; learning through reflection and reflecting on learning will enhance future work. Keeping a reflective clinical notebook has been a key component throughout your project. At each stage of proposal writing, as you have made choices that further directed your work, you have addressed the basic questions of what, so what, and now what. Now, as you finish your project, reflecting on the full process and product provides the opportunity to cement learning and gain a basis for future ideas and plans. Prompts to guide reflections on your project work include the following:

1. Why was this work important to you?
2. What was the most important thing that you learned from creating this proposal and project?
3. How does this proposal and project help you document what you do as an advanced clinician?
4. What was it like for you to create this proposal and project? What most surprised you about your work on this proposal?
5. What did you gain from creating this proposal and project? What new skills or strategies were acquired?
6. How did this proposal and project expand your previous knowledge? How did this advance your thinking about the topic or subject area?
7. How did this work enhance your role as an advanced clinician?
8. How will you be able to use what you gained from this experience in future work as an advanced clinician?
9. If you were to continue your work on this product, what further approaches would you consider?
10. What further learning goals do you have related to this work?

## REFERENCES

American Association of Colleges of Nursing. (2015). *The doctor of nursing practice: Current issues and clarifying recommendations.* https://www.aacnnursing.org/Portals/42/DNP/DNP-Implementation.pdf

American Association of Colleges of Nursing. (2021). *The essentials.* https://www.aacnnursing.org/essentials

Boyer, E. L. (1990). *Scholarship reconsidered: Priorities of the professoriate.* Carnegie Foundation for the Advancement of Teaching.

Cronenwett, L., Sherwood, G., Pohl, J., Barnsteiner, J., Moore, S., Sullivan, D. T., Ward, D., & Warren, J. (2009). Quality and safety education for advanced nursing practice. *Nursing Outlook, 57*(6), 338–348. https://doi.org/10.1016/j.outlook.2009.07.009

Huber, M., & Hutchings, P. (2005). *The advancement of learning: Building the teaching commons.* Jossey-Bass.

Institute of Medicine. (2003). *Health professions education: A bridge to quality.* National Academies Press.

Interprofessional Education Collaborative. (2011). *Core competencies for interprofessional collaborative practice.* https://ipec.memberclicks.net/assets/2011-Original.pdf

Oermann, M., & Hays, H. (2018). *Writing for publication in nursing* (4th ed.). Springer Publishing Company.

# Appendix A. Clinical Project Triangle

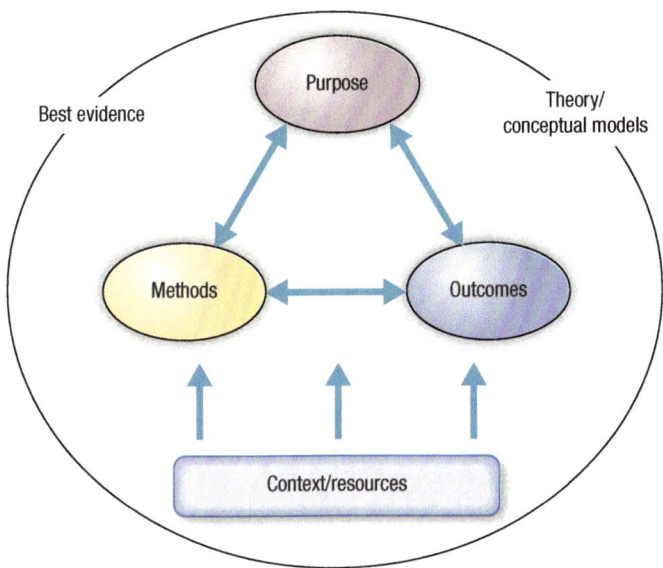

Once you have clearly identified the project problem, you are ready to use the components of this model to develop your proposal. The checklist in Appendix B assists you in reflecting on your work.

# Appendix B. Checklist for Planning or Self-Assessment of a Specific Project

As you move forward with your project proposal, check to see whether you have adequately addressed each of the following. Indicate "agree" or "disagree" to confirm that each area has been thoroughly considered. As you move toward proposal completion, do a reflective review or critique of its strengths and weaknesses. What are points you can strengthen?

| Concept | Have You Considered | Agree/Disagree |
|---|---|---|
| Evidence-based practice | What evidence is available to guide initiating and implementing a particular project? | |
| Theory or conceptual model | What theory or model might best guide the project? | |
| Logistics/context with assessment of unit/setting | Have you assessed the need for your project and confirmed with clinical agency staff? Have you assessed the feasibility of your project? What are the facilitators/barriers for completing the project in a specific setting with a specific population? | |
| Purpose | Does the purpose flow from the identified problem? What is to be achieved with the project? | |
| Methods | Have you considered diverse potential approaches to address your problem? What is the best approach to your given problem and project purpose? | |
| Outcomes evaluation | What project outcomes are to be evaluated? How will you know your project is successful? | |

# Appendix C. Proposal Abstract: "Improving the Care of Patients With Chronic Kidney Disease Using Evidence-Based Guidelines"

*Gwenyth Wagner*

## PROBLEM STATEMENT

There is a documented gap between best-evidence guidelines and implementation of these guidelines in the care of chronic kidney disease (CKD) patients in primary care.

## PURPOSE

To develop and implement a quality improvement survey to evaluate adherence to clinical guidelines for the care of patients with CKD and ultimately suggest approaches to improve translation of evidence-based care into practice.

## CONTEXT

The setting will be a Midwestern primary care clinic.

## METHODS

- A quality-improvement tool will be developed from best-evidence literature to gain practice-level clinical performance data.

- Clinical performance measures will be derived from the *Kidney Disease Outcomes Quality Initiative* guidelines.

- A chart review of approximately 50 patients with a glomerular filtration rate <60 mL/min/1.73 m$^2$ will be conducted using the clinical performance tool.

- A talking-points summary will be developed to share the best-practice guidelines, results of the chart review, and an evaluation of the quality-improvement tool with the medical director and other staff. Practice improvement steps will be generated.

# Appendix D. Proposal Abstract: "Improving Diabetes Care Delivery in an Integrated Health Clinic"

*Jane Robinson*

Populations with serious mental illness are often underserved and likely to have barriers to accessing primary care services. When these patients do seek primary care, the result is often fragmented and communication among multiple providers lacks efficiency and coordination. A co-located primary care clinic was recently established in a large behavioral health setting to improve access to primary care for this population. Prior to opening the clinic, in a survey of 499 client respondents, 82 indicated they needed help managing their diabetes. Multiple providers with varied backgrounds are providing care in the new clinic setting where potential gaps in the delivery of diabetes-related care are likely. The purpose of this project is to evaluate the care provided to patients with type 2 diabetes mellitus in the primary care clinic by multiple providers compared to a standard. The standard will be medical care for diabetes management according to the current American Diabetes Association (ADA) guidelines. A retrospective chart review using a standards checklist based on the ADA guidelines will be used to evaluate care provided by a number of different providers. The intent is to identify any gaps in care. Feedback will be shared with providers in a post-study discussion. Improvement implications may include the potential for enhanced documentation and use of the ADA standards checklist as a tool to improve delivery of care.

# Appendix E. Project Abstract: "Unit-Based Council Chairs' Perception of Unit-Based Councils"

*Sonya Curtis*

## BACKGROUND

Nurse managers are consistently dealing with day-to-day operational management of the microsystem for which they are held accountable and responsible. Nurse managers are not always visible on their units or at the points of care so may not know the patients' needs in maintaining the plan of care that has been determined. Staff nurses verbalize frustrations with their lack of autonomy regarding decision-making at the bedside and helping to change current professional clinical practice. This critical problem is impacting nurse job satisfaction, intent to leave, and patient care. Literature encourages leaders to collaborate with staff nurses to create work environments that maximize their ability to provide optimal care to patients. The literature suggests introducing an element of shared governance, considered for this project to be a unit-based council (UBC).

## PURPOSE

The purpose of this quality-improvement (QI) project was to evaluate UBC chairs' perception of UBCs.

## METHOD

This QI project surveyed a sample of 37 RNs, who are UBC chairs, from a large Midwestern academic medical center. The UBC Perceptions Survey, consisting of five open-ended questions, assessed broadly the UBC chairs' perception of the functioning of their UBC. The UBCs Functionality Measurement Tool (21 items allowing for agreement/disagreement about characteristics of successful UBCs) was utilized to evaluate more directly the perception of UBCs' functioning.

## FINDINGS AND CONCLUSIONS

A majority of respondents ($N = 29/37$) reported the UBCs to be high functioning. Qualitative themes supported participants' appreciation of the UBC, including themes of valuing the UBC, improving patient outcomes, feeling appreciated, improving nursing practice, and having a voice. Aggregate data from surveys were used to provide feedback to the UBC chairs with the goal of ongoing QI related to UBCs. Project findings support the value of UBCs in hospital practice and decision-making for nurses participating in UBCs at the point of care.

# Appendix F. Proposal Abstract: "Descriptive Evidence Generating: Learning From Practitioner Owners of Clinics"

*Paula Israel*

## BACKGROUND

In Missouri, a collaborative practice agreement is required for NPs to deliver care. Delegated tasks are more restrictive than what is possible based on education and scope of practice granted to NPs by the state board of nursing. In addition, limitations are imposed by legislators.

## SIGNIFICANCE

A dearth of medical providers has created unprecedented opportunities for NPs. Existing literature cites limited autonomy, reduced rates of reimbursement, incongruent state practice acts, and lack of business acumen as barriers to independent NP clinic ownership. NPs are identified as one viable solution to the lack of primary care providers in the United States.

## PURPOSE

Opportunities and barriers to NPs working collaboratively with physicians in NP-owned clinics will be explored through the review of the literature and by description of experiences of NP clinic owners in one Midwestern state.

## THEORY

The systems theory of structure, process, and outcomes provides a framework for this project. Regulations and reimbursement (structure) allowing NPs to practice to the full extent of their training (process) could increase healthcare access (outcome) for patients.

## METHODS

This will be a descriptive, exploratory study of NP clinic owners. An online survey, consisting of 11 open-ended and four structured questions, was developed from the literature and insights gained from observing one business owner's patterns and practices. Fourteen of 19 identified clinic owners will meet inclusion criteria and be invited to describe their experience through this self-report.

## ANALYSIS

Descriptive analysis will include a summary of participant characteristics. Content analysis of qualitative data responses will be completed seeking key themes. Implications for practice, policy, education, and research will be generated from the findings.

# Appendix G. Proposal Abstract: "Evidence Synthesis Plus: Anesthesia Considerations and Implications for Obese Pediatric Patients"

Karri Arndt

The number of Americans classified as overweight or obese has been increasing at an alarming rate over the past 30 years. Overweight and obesity in both children and adults have been identified not only by the U.S. Department of Health and Human Services, Centers for Disease Control and Prevention as an epidemic in the United States, but also as a pandemic by the World Health Organization (WHO). The WHO considers childhood obesity as one of the most serious public health challenges of the 21st century. As the rate of overweight and obese individuals increases, so does the economic burden of obesity-related healthcare in the United States and worldwide.

Ambulatory surgery centers are also seeing a greater number of obese pediatric patients in their facilities for what are typically considered minor to moderate outpatient procedures. However, the presence of these comorbid conditions is making safe care a challenge in these facilities as anesthesia providers do not have the same ancillary resources, invasive equipment, difficult-airway devices, or various medical services readily available in the event of a complication or emergency. These facilities also are not equipped for overnight stays should perioperative complications arise. It is imperative that anesthesia providers have a thorough understanding of the anesthetic implications and unique challenges associated with the obese pediatric population.

The purpose of this project is to review the current literature related to perioperative morbidity, mortality, issues, and concerns that arise when caring for obese pediatric patients requiring anesthesia services and to prepare an educational resource and an article for potential publication.

Current evidence-based data will describe the prevalence of obesity in children, identify coexisting diseases and their management, discuss pharmacokinetic and pharmacodynamic considerations, identify anesthetic management techniques for this unique patient population, and identify specific questions that require further research. The intent is to increase awareness of pediatric obesity and its implications and to improve knowledge and competency of anesthesia providers, which will better prepare them to safely handle increasing numbers of obese children, especially in the ambulatory setting.

## METHODOLOGY

The methodology for collecting data and information for this project will include a systematic review of the literature from PubMed and the Cumulative Index to Nursing and Allied Health Literature (CINAHL) using the key terms: *pediatric*, *obesity*, *anesthesia*, *morbidity*, and *mortality*. Other sources to be searched include the American Society of Anesthesiologists, the American Association of Nurse Anesthetists, the Society for Pediatric Anesthesia, and current anesthesia text and reference books, using the same key-word searches. The CDC will be searched for current statistical data related to the prevalence of and trends in childhood obesity.

Information obtained from the database searches will be reviewed and critically assessed for relevance and reliability. References in high-quality studies will also be reviewed for potential relevant material. Obtained data will then be organized in an easy-to-review database matrix that will identify the reference citation, type of article or research conducted, evidence obtained, key points, and limitations. Information will then be combined into a concise educational resource and review article for submission for publication. These resources will provide a literature synthesis with discussion of state-of-the-art information, summary of the anesthetic implications associated with the perioperative care of obese pediatric patients, and recommendations for future research.

# Appendix H. Proposal Abstract: "Evidence-Based Quality Improvement: Improving the Communication of Clinical Information Between Nurses and Physicians in Long-Term Care"

*Linda Kroeger*

Based on personal observation; experience in receiving calls from long-term care (LTC) facilities; and conversations with physicians, RNs, and LPNs who expressed frustration with their phone interactions, a brief needs-assessment was done regarding nurse/provider calls to and from LTC facilities. Several LPNs reported that their biggest fear was calling to speak with a physician regarding a change in a patient's condition because they lacked confidence in their ability to answer questions asked by the physician.

## PURPOSE

The purpose of this quality-improvement (QI) project is to use developed methods, established protocols, and structured communication techniques to develop and implement a program to teach LTC nurses, including RNs and LPNs, how to efficiently and competently collect and communicate clinical information to physicians.

## SETTING

A request for participation in this QI project will be made to the director of nursing of a local nursing home. The nursing home consists of six units; each unit has 16 beds and the facility capacity is 96 residents. The facility provides long-term residential care and skilled nursing care.

## SAMPLE

The nursing staff at this LTC facility is composed of RNs and LPNs. RNs include the director of nursing, the assistant director of nursing, and two Minimum Data Set nurses.

An RN and two LPNs staff the LTC unit on the day and evening shifts, and two LPNs are responsible for the night shift. The nursing home also has nurses who work on call and other LPNs available. The number of RNs and LPNs who will be invited to participate in this QI program for communication training is approximately 13.

## QUALITY IMPROVEMENT PLAN

The training program for communication techniques was developed from evidence-based practices. It will begin with an introduction on organizing tips to consider before calling the physician. This will be followed by instruction on the use of the situation, background, assessment, recommendation (SBAR) communication technique. The SBAR method has the support of the Institute for Healthcare Improvement and The Joint Commission. As described by the American Medical Directors Association (AMDA), the SBAR is an established, evidence-based method shown to be effective in improving clinical communication skills. This part of the training program will be made into a PowerPoint presentation with a voiceover that could be used for future staff development training programs. Protocol cards, developed by AMDA for use by LTC nurses, are designed to facilitate the gathering and presentation of information during physician phone calls. The 15 most common clinical problems, for example, pain and agitation, and their protocol cards, will be included in a handout. The AMDA protocol cards will be reviewed, and an example using one card to evaluate a clinical problem will be demonstrated. A survey measuring nurse satisfaction with telephone communication (10 items) will be administered to LTC nurses before the program, immediately after the program, and 4 to 6 weeks after instruction. A Wilcoxon signed-rank test will be used to assess for satisfaction score differences on telephone communication.

# Index

AACN. *See* American Association of Colleges of Nursing
abstract
   preparations, considerations for, 143
   proposal
      as tool 137
Agency for Healthcare Research and Quality (AHRQ) 129
AGREE. *See* Appraisal of Guidelines for Research and Evaluations
AHRQ. *See* Agency for Healthcare Research and Quality
AI. *See* artificial intelligence
American Association of Colleges of Nursing (AACN), 3, 4, 27, 53, 77
American Psychological Association (APA), 111
analysis of variance (ANOVA) 106
ANOVA. *See* analysis of variance
APA. *See* American Psychological Association
Appraisal of Guidelines for Research and Evaluations (AGREE), 40
artificial intelligence (AI), 115
audit trail, 97

big-picture tools and problem-solving strategies, 13–14
broad writing plan, 12–13

CINAHL. *See* Cumulative Index to Nursing and Allied Health Literature
CITI. *See* Collaborative Institutional Training Initiative
clinical application scholarship
   benefits of reflection, 5
   competency-based approach, 3–4; *see also* practice scholarship applications
   documenting scholarship, framework for, 3–4
   proposal writing for, 4
   reflective self-assessments, 4
   seeking and gaining mentor, 7
clinical project proposal
   checklist, 7, 8
   clinical application scholarship, 3–4
   clinical problems
      advice from DNP students, 24
      area of concern, 19–20
      bringing ideas into shape, 21
      challenges with, 23
      clinical practicum work and clinical mentors, 20
      context description and setting boundaries, 22
      development/write-up, thinking during, 22
      fine-tuning, problem statement, 23
      literature review, 35–42
      narrowing the topic, 21–22
      peer review of, 23–24
      problem name and description clarification, 22
      problem significance, 23
      project triangle, 24
      quality improvement, 27–32

   common terms related to, 6–7
   mapping out, 77
   method section, 85–92
   project triangle, 7
   reflective clinician, reviewing best evidence, 6
   scholarly, 5–6
   writing, 4–5
clinical scholarship, 142
   caring for self, 145
   developing and continuing the mentor partnership, 145
   models, 141–142
   national priorities, 142
Collaborative Institutional Training Initiative (CITI), 113
Common Rule, 113
concept-mapping tools, 13
conflict of interest, 112–113
Cronbach's alpha, 97
Cumulative Index to Nursing and Allied Health Literature (CINAHL), 38

data-analysis plans
   advice from DNP students, 108
   for analyzing data, 104
   correct inferential tests 106
   descriptive data, sample characteristics plans for, 105
   for organizing data, 103–104
   for project completion, 108–109
   project triangle, 104
   quick tips, 107–108
   for reporting, 106–108
   reporting the data-analysis results, visual presentation, 106–107
   sample frequency count, 105–107
   sharing qualitative results plans, 105
   visualization, 104
data collection
   comments on, 89–90
   advice from DNP students, 99
   detailed plan for, 95–96
   examples
      descriptive evidence generation, 90
      evidence-based quality improvement, 90
   further challenges
      instrument development, 99
      project internal validity, 99
   other considerations
      data organization, 98
      setting for, 98
      storing data, 98
      technology and, 99
      timeline, 98–99
pilot testing, implementation, 130
qualitative context, 87–88
quantitative context, 88

data collection (*cont.*)
   setting and sample considerations, 90–91
   strategies for
      interviews and surveys, 88–89
      observation, 89
      planning for, 89
      record/document reviews, 89
      written surveys, 89
   tools for, 87, 96–98
      credibility issues, 97
      pilot test of tools, 98
      protocol procedure, 97–98
      reliability and validity, 96–97
      thorough description sharing, 96
data organization, 98
decision trails, 14
   final protocol implementation, 131
drafting, 13

edit-and-revise process, 137–138
Education Resources Information Center (ERIC), 38
EHR. *See* electronic health records
electronic health records (EHRs), 88, 105
ERIC. *See* Education Resources Information Center
*Essentials. See* practice scholarship applications
ethical issues
   artificial intelligence (AI), 115
   avoiding plagiarism, 112
   conflict of interest, 112–113
   data integrity, use, 114–115
   diversity and inclusion, 113–114
   final steps, 115
   human subjects, institutional review boards, 113, 114
   permission to use instruments, 112
   professionalism, 111–112
evidence gaining
   challenges/facilitators
      decision trail, 39–40
      issues and limitations, 39
   organization
      archiving and cataloguing, 41
      documenting sources, 42
      final touches to, 41–42
      reference matrix, 41
      reference matrix format, 41
   reading and critiquing
      approaches regarding, 40
      quality of, 40–41
evidence-based practice, 6
evidence-based project
   descriptive evidence-generating approaches, 81
   evidence-based quality improvement approaches, 80–81
evidence synthesis plus approaches, 80–81

feasibility of project, 82
final project write-up 138
final proposal
   appendices, 118
   proposal structure, 118
   proposal substance, 118
   self-editing, 118
   writing, editing, 118
final report, 135–138
   abstract as a tool, 137
   addressing project strengths and limits, 137
   discussion section, 136–137
   edit-and-revise process, 137–138
   final project write-up, 138
   from idea to completed project, 135–136
   identifying implications, 137
   initial literature review, 137
   introduction and method sections, 136
   literature review, 136
   planning to present, 138
   project notebook, 138
   relating findings, purpose statement, 136
   results section, 136
fishbone-type diagram, 14
focused descriptive report, 31
formal systematic reviews, 37–38
free writing, 14

Google Scholar, 38

information literacy, 37
institutional review boards (IRBs), 113
interviews
   strategies for data collection, 88–89
IRBs. *See* institutional review boards

literature review
   advice from DNP students, 39
   beginning, 37
   challenges/facilitators, 39–40
   formal, 37–38
   literature search, 38–39
   multiple approaches for, 36
   organization, 41–42
      archiving and cataloguing, 41
      documenting sources, 42
      final touches to, 41–42
      reference matrix, 41
      reference matrix format, 41
   synthesis
      checklist for, 48
      individual article description, 46–47
      introductory overview, 49
      introductory section to, 48–49
      matrix articles, critique of, 46–47
      organizing approaches, 47–48
      prewriting, 48
      reference matrix, findings, 47
      reviewing and critiquing, reference matrix, 46
      summary statements, 49
      systematic literature review methods, 49
      tips to consider, 50
      translating evidence, 49–50
      uses for, 49

tips for getting started, 42
type of, 37
literature search
  databases, 38
  evidence gaining (*See* evidence gaining)
  inclusion/exclusion criteria, 38
  key words, 38
  practical and methodological screens, 38
  primary/secondary sources, 38–39
literature synthesis
  checklist for, 49
  individual article description, 46–47
  introductory overview, 49
  introductory section to, 48–49
  matrix articles, critique of, 46–47
  organizing approaches, 47–48
  prewriting, 48
  reference matrix
    findings, 47
    reviewing and critiquing, 46
  summary statements
    concept definitions or populations, variations in, 47
    main/relevant concepts/themes, 47
    methods quality, 47–48
  systematic literature review methods, 49
  tips to consider, 50
  translating evidence, 49–50
  uses for, 49

mentors, formal reviews seeking, 15
methodological screens, 38
method section
  advice from DNP students, 92
  common approaches, writing up methods, 91–92
  data collection
    comments on, 89–90
    descriptive evidence generation, 90
    evidence-based quality improvement, 90
    examples, 90
    interviews and surveys, 88–89
    observation, 89
    planning for, 89
    qualitative context, 87–88
    quantitative context, 88
    record/document reviews, 89
    setting and sample considerations, 90–91
    strategies for, 88–89
    tools, 87
    written surveys, 89
  focusing methods, 86–87
  importance of, 85–86
  selecting approaches, 91
  setting and sample considerations, 90–91

National Database of Nursing Quality Indicators, 99

observations, 89
one-page early reflection, 14
ongoing reflective journaling, 14

outcomes evaluation
  accessibility, considerations for, 65
  clinical unit policies, 67
  evaluation principles, 67
  identifying, 64
  naming, 63–65
  other considerations, 66
  project triangle, 65
  purpose statements/aims, 64
  "so what" factor, addressing, 66
  systems models and
    backward design, 65
    outcomes context, describing, 64
  technology and outcomes data, 66
  timelines for, 65–66
  tips for getting started, 67
outlining, 14

peer reviews, 15
  problem statements, 23–24
  proposal draft, 119
  purpose statement, 73
PICOT. *See* Population, Intervention, Comparison, Outcomes, and Time questions
plagiarism, 112
plan-do-check-act (PDCA), 56
Population, Intervention, Comparison, Outcomes, and Time (PICOT) questions, 71
practice scholarship applications
  *Essentials*, 9, 16, 24, 32, 42, 50, 58, 67, 73, 83, 92, 99, 108, 115, 122, 132, 138, 145
practical screen, 38
Preferred Reporting Items for Systematic Reviews and Meta-Analyses (PRISMA), 40–41
prewriting, 12, 48
PRISMA. *See* Preferred Reporting Items for Systematic Reviews and Meta-Analyses
problem, population, change, outcome (PPCO) question, 71
problem-solving and concept mapping, 14
problem-solving question prompts, 14
problem statements
  challenges with, 23
  fine-tuning, 23
  peer review of, 23–24
  problem significance, 23
  project triangle, 24
professionalism, 111–112
project charter, 4–5
project management
  engaging the team, 130
  pilot testing, implementation, 130
  professional communication with team members, 130–131
  revisiting project evaluation data, 130
  scheduling specific project components, 130
project mapping
  advice from DNP students, 83
  common challenges, 82
  descriptive evidence-generating approaches, 81
  designing, 77

project mapping (*cont.*)
    evidence synthesis plus approaches, 80–81
    evidence-based approaches, 78, 80
    evidence-based project visual organizer, 78, 79
    evidence-based quality-improvement approaches, 80
    further considerations for, 81–82
    project triangle, 78–80
    sample project using organizing template, 78, 79
    project mentor, 7
project notebooks, 15–16, 138; *see also* practice scholarship applications
project presentation
    abstract preparations, considerations for, 143
    career portfolio, 144
    career, role transitions, 145
    clinical projects proposals for, 144
    formats, 142–143
    further mapping out, 145
    planning for publication, 144
    for poster presentations, 143
    proposals, grant writing, 144
    verbal, 143
    wrapping up, 144
project triangle, 147
    advice from DNP students, 24
    data-analysis plans 104
    mapping in, 78–80
    problem statements, 24
proposal draft, 117–121
    budget finalizing, 119
    final proposal
        appendices, 118
        self-editing, 118
        structure, 118
        substance, 118
    finalizing timeline, 119
    further writing tips, 118–119
    project implementation and final report write-up, 120–122
    reflecting, self-editing, 120
    revising, first draft, 118
    sample format for power point presentation of, 120, 121
    tools to facilitate completion, 119–120
        decision trail, 120
        peer review, 119
        project team and committee, 119
        self-review, 120
proposals
    clear communication, 6
    clinical problems
        challenges with, 23
        fine-tuning, problem statement, 23
        peer review of, 23–24
        problem significance, 23
        project triangle, 24
    clinical scholarship models, 141–142
    national priorities, 142
PubMed, 38
purpose statement
    advice from DNP students, 73
    checklist for, 72–73
    clinical problem relationship, 70
    clinical question, using, 71
    evidence-based protocols for, 70
    final purpose statement, 72
    peer review of, 73
    from problem to solution, 70–71
    project triangle, 70
    revising, 71–72
    semantics and, 69–70

QSEN. *See* quality and safety education for nurses
quality improvement (QI) projects
    examples, 29
    implementation, 129–130
        adhering to project procedures, 129
        assumptions in, 128–129
        continuing professional communication with team members, 130
        data-collection procedures, 130
        engaging the team, 130
        final protocol, 131–132
        issues in, 129
        pilot testing the implementation, 130
        project management, 129–131
        revisiting project evaluation data, 130
        revisiting, proposal protocol, 129
        scheduling specific project components, 130
    populations perspectives, 29
    practical perspective, 28
    problem solving
        checklists as, 31
        documentation, 30
        focused descriptive report sharing, 31
        needs assessments, 30
        root cause analysis, 30–31
        SWOT analyses, 30–32
        technology and large data sets, 31
    scholarship definition, 4
    systems perspectives, 28–29
    written proposal, 11–12
quality and safety education for nurses (QSEN), 142

rapid critical appraisal (RCA), 40
RCA. *See* rapid critical appraisal
reflection, benefits of, 5
reference matrix format, 41
research utilization, 6

scholarly dialogue, 5
scholarly proposals, 5–6
scholarly writing, 5
    drafting, 13
    with reading, 12
    strategies to, 13–15
        big-picture tools, 13–14
        one-page early reflection, 14
        ongoing reflective journaling, 14
        peer and mentor reviews, 15
        reflective-writing strategies, 14

self-editing, 15
tools to help document, 14–15
tips to maintain momentum for, 12–13
tools for, 12
self-editing, 15
self-plagiarism, 112
structured questions, 14

theoretical/conceptual model frameworks
advice from DNP students, 58
appropriate, selection of, 55–56
boundaries, 54
concepts definition, 54, 55
consistency, 55
efficiency, 55
organization, 55
sample project topics and theories, 56–58
structure and relationships, 54–55
translation of evidence, 6

triangulation, 89, 97
Typhon, 31

Watson's caring theory, 96
written surveys, 89
writing plans
big-picture tools, 13–14
drafting, 13
one-page early reflection, 14
ongoing reflective journaling, 14
peer and mentor reviews, 15
project notebook, to document, 15–16
with reading, 12
reflective-writing strategies, 14
self-directed, 12–13
self-editing, 15
as tool, 12
tools to help document, 14–15
writing prompts, 14